The Periodic Paralysis Guide And Workbook:
Be The Best You Can Be *Naturally*

About the Authors

Calvin and Susan Q. Knittle-Hunter are the co-creators, co-founders and co-directors of the Periodic Paralysis Network, Inc. (PPNI), an independent, educational corporation, designed to provide support, education and advocacy to individuals with Periodic Paralysis (PP).

Calvin, the Primary Director of PPNI, earned B.S. degrees in Behavioral Science and Psychology at Westminster College and the University of Utah. He also holds an M.Ed. degree in Special Education and M.S. degree in Information Technology from the University of Utah and Capella University. Calvin worked in a variety of fields including teaching, corrections and case management.

Susan, the Managing Director of PPNI, earned B.S. degrees in Psychology and Special Education at the University of Utah and spent many years as a teacher and case manager working with children and adults with disabilities. She suffers from a rare and disabling mineral metabolic disorder called Periodic Paralysis.

Calvin and Susan have co-authored and co-published three books; *living with Periodic Paralysis: The Mystery Unraveled, Sotos Syndrome: A Tribute to Sandy* and *Moments In Time: At Home In The Woods*.

Calvin and Susan are retired special education teachers living on the Olympic Peninsula in Washington with their spoiled cat Jasmine where they are presently writing their next books. In their spare time, Calvin tends their organic garden and Susan enjoys genealogy research.

The Periodic Paralysis Guide And Workbook:
Be The Best You Can Be *Naturally*

Susan Quentine Knittle-Hunter

&

Calvin Hunter

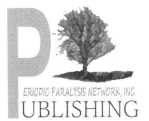

Periodic Paralysis Network, Inc. Publishing
Sequim, Washington U.S.A.
2014

The Periodic Paralysis Guide And Workbook:
Be The Best You Can Be Naturally

Susan Q. Knittle-Hunter
B. S. Special Education
B. S. Psychology
&
Calvin Hunter
M.S. Information Technology
M. Ed. Special Education
B.S. Psychology
B.S. Behavioral Science

Periodic Paralysis Network, Inc Publishing
Sequim, Washington U.S.A.

All rights reserved. No part of the book may be reproduced or transmitted in any form or by any means, electronic or mechanical, including photocopying, recording or by any information storage or retrieval system, without written permission from the authors, except for the inclusion of brief quotations in a review.

Copyright © 2014
Library of Congress Cataloging-in-Publication Data:
The Periodic Paralysis Guide And Workbook: Be The Best You Can Be Naturally

Susan Q. Knittle-Hunter
&
Calvin Hunter

First Edition
ISBN-13:
978-1503253810

ISBN-10:
1503253813

1. Andersen-Tawil Syndrome 2. Periodic Paralysis 3. Hypokalemia 4. Hyperkalemia 5. Normokalemia 6. Hypokalemic Periodic Paralysis 7. Hyperkalemic Periodic Paralysis 8. Medical Malpractice 9. Rare Diseases 10. Potassium Channel Myopathies 11. Inspiration 12. Muscular Dystrophy 13. Voltage-Gated Potassium Ion Channel 14. Ion Channelopathies 15. Self-Help 16. Mineral Metabolic Disorders 17. Metabolic Acidosis 18. Paramyotonia Congenita

Printed in the United States of America.
2014

Notice-Disclaimer

The ideas in this book are based on the authors' personal experiences with Periodic Paralysis, and as such are intended to provide only educational information on the covered subject to the reader. This book should not be used as a medical manual nor should this book be used as a diagnostic tool for Periodic Paralysis. The reader should consult a qualified health care professional or physician with expertise in Periodic Paralysis.

Dedication

This workbook is dedicated to the members of our Periodic Paralysis Network Education, Support and Advocacy Discussion Group who inspire and support me every day.

Also by Susan Q. Knittle-Hunter & Calvin Hunter

living with Periodic Paralysis: The Mystery Unraveled

Also by Susan Q. Knittle-Hunter

Sotos Syndrome: A tribute To Sandy

Also by Calvin Hunter

Moments In Time: At Home In The Woods

Table Of Contents

	Acknowledgments	viii
	Preface	ix
	Introduction	xi

Section I: The Facts

	Getting Started	1
One	Periodic Paralysis: The Basic Facts	5
Two	The Periodic Paralyses: More Detail	9
Three	An Ion Channelopathy: A Mineral Metabolic Disorder	17
Four	Possible Complications: The Most Common	19
Five	More Complications: Understanding The Complexity	35

Section II: The Plan

Six	The Plan: The Outline	45
Seven	Educate Yourself: Discussion Groups, Websites, Internet and Books	49
Eight	Describe Your Episodes: Paralysis Accompanying Symptoms	53
Nine	Monitor Your Vitals: Tools For The Job	59
Ten	Identify And Eliminate Triggers: Avoid-Chart-Journal-Monitor	71
Eleven	Relieve Your Symptoms: Changing Lives Naturally	87
Twelve	Find A Doctor Who Cares: Not Easy But Possible	109
Thirteen	Get A Diagnosis: Hit Them With The Facts	115
Fourteen	Get Proper Medical Treatment: Assemble And Direct The Team	127
Fifteen	Direct The Paramedics And EMT's: No IV's Please	131
Sixteen	Direct The ER And Hospital Staff: Avoid The Pitfalls	135
Seventeen	Prognosis: The Best You Can Be	139
Eighteen	The Conclusion: Hope	141

Section III: The Journal

Nineteen	The Personal Periodic Paralysis Journal: Put It Together	145
	Index	191

Acknowledgments

As in my previous book, I would like to thank my late mother Lahlee Duggins for showing me how to handle adversity, illness, pain and disability with dignity, bravery and a sense of humor. To my late father William J. Knittle, thank you for your unconditional love, understanding and support. Thanks to my husband, Calvin, for saving my life and all you do to keep me alive and for your love, patience, and caring. Thank you also for your never-ending research and for your help with formatting and editing of this book. Thank you Julie for taking care of me and for wiping my tears when I could not. I want to thank Rosie, my therapist, for your constant faith and support and believing us when no one else did. Thank you Laurel, my lab technician, for your special help, understanding and support by coming out to the car to take my blood at those critical times I was in paralysis and for your professional advice and friendship. I have a special thanks for the staff at Lincare in Grants Pass, Oregon, especially Carol and Tim, for saving my life by listening when no one else would, for going the extra mile. I would like to thank the neurologist, cardiologist and renal specialist who believed me and finally diagnosed me. To the doctors and medical professionals who believed me and now see me and learn from us about Periodic Paralysis, thank you. For my children Tammy, Jeff and Shari and her husband Tom, thank you for your love and understanding and for being available for me always. Thanks also to my brother, Brud, for your love and understanding. I am so sorry we share this disease. Thank you cousin Linda for all of the information you provided me about your father, my uncle that helped in my diagnosis. Also thanks to a few of my family members for sharing medical information with me as I traced our medical genealogy, especially my cousin Shari. Finally, thanks to the few family members who believe me and support me. Lastly, thank you to the members of our Periodic Paralysis Network Support, Education and Advocacy Group who give me support, validation and inspiration each and everyday.

Preface

A preface for a book is written to explain what the book is about, why the author wrote the book, why it is important, where the idea for the book originated, how it came to be and how long it took to write. With this in mind, I will begin by explaining that this book is about a very rare, hereditary, and debilitating mineral metabolic disorder, with which I have been diagnosed, called Periodic Paralysis (PP). It is the second book written specifically about this relatively unknown condition. My husband Calvin and I previously wrote, *living with Periodic Paralysis: The Mystery Unraveled,* based on our own experiences and research. In it we tell our story, provide information about Periodic Paralysis not found anywhere else, and deliver ideas about how to better manage symptoms and discuss the psychological and social aspects of living with the condition.

The idea for a second book came from the need, of a user-friendly workbook and guide to assist individuals with this condition to be the best they can be by using the natural and common sense methods as outlined in the first book. This is important because very little information exists about how to treat the symptoms of Periodic Paralysis, other than the use of off-label drugs, which can be harmful to many individuals or are not tolerated well. The idea for this book originated from our own experiences, study and experimentation and the need of others who suffer from this condition. This book actually took more than four years to compile and write.

We know this need exists because Calvin and I interact daily with over 300 very ill individuals, from around the world, who are members in our Periodic Paralysis Network Support, Education and Advocacy Group and others who contact us by email through our PPN Website, our PPN Facebook Pages, our PPN Blog or through searching for us after reading our first book. These individuals, their families and caregivers, and several new members each week, need assistance and we spend our days providing support, education, advocacy, validation and hope in an otherwise hopeless world for them.

They are attempting to find the names of specialists who can help them and diagnose them and seeking a simple pill or medication to stop the paralysis and other cruel 'quality of life stealing' symptoms plaguing them daily. The truth is there are very few "specialists" or doctors in the world who know about or fully understand all aspects of the many forms of Periodic Paralysis. There is no simple pill or drug; no magic cure for Periodic Paralysis. Most doctors do not recognize Periodic Paralysis and genetic testing is nearly non-existent for most forms and therefore they will not diagnose their patients or will diagnose them with somatic disorders. However, when these individuals come to our forum, we are able to provide them with hope and methods to assist them to find a doctor who cares and to get a diagnosis based on their symptoms. We also provide methods to assist them to relieve their symptoms in natural ways. We help them to improve their lives with the information and methods we have learned and I practice everyday.

Through this new guide, workbook and journal, we have included all of these ideas and the tools to be successful. We want to empower individuals with Periodic Paralysis by providing a hands-on, user-friendly implement in one handbook with a series of plans made up life changing goals and objectives. These are expanded from the first book as well as the simple and easy to follow instructions to carry them out. *The Periodic*

Paralysis Guide And Workbook: Be The Best You Can Be Naturally, offers HOPE to everyone with Periodic Paralysis, in the same manner as our book, *living with Periodic Paralysis: The Mystery Unraveled.*

In conclusion, we are aware that it is not an easy path in life for individuals with Periodic Paralysis. We know we must constantly balance on an ever-changing tightrope. We are not able to provide anyone who has Periodic Paralysis with a cure or a magic drug. We cannot diagnose anyone or suggest a specialist who can help. However, we do know that through this hands on and user-friendly guide and workbook, we can give others hope through the knowledge we share, the ideas we pass along in all areas of dealing with and managing their symptoms and with validation and support. We wrote this second book about Periodic Paralysis, to give hope to others who suffer with this condition and to guide them to be the best they can be naturally.

Introduction

This book will provide readers with information and methods to better manage the often over-whelming and disabling symptoms of all forms of Periodic Paralysis. *The Periodic Paralysis Guide And Workbook: Be The Best You Can Be Naturally*, is the second book written specifically about Periodic Paralysis, a very rare, usually inherited and often debilitating mineral metabolic disorder. It contains comprehensive information about the various forms of the condition written in an easy to understand format. It is a user-friendly guide, a set of plans, instructions and ideas for aiding individuals with all forms of Periodic Paralysis, to better manage their symptoms in natural and common sense methods. It is a workbook with a set of tools such as charts, forms and even a medical journal, with clear instructions for completing and using them. Each is designed to be individualized and may be utilized for the various plans or sections of the book. The charts and forms may be scanned and used separately or the pages may simply be completed in the book itself for keeping all medical information in one place. Easily transportable, this book is also a handbook and can accompany each visit to doctor appointments, the ER or the hospital. This guide may stand-alone or may be used in conjunction with the first book about Periodic Paralysis, *living with Periodic Paralysis: The Mystery Unraveled*. This guide, workbook and handbook is designed to assist individuals with all forms of Periodic Paralysis to 'be the best they can be naturally.'

Section I
The Facts

Getting Started

In order to get started with this guide and workbook, we first need to take a look back at our book, *living with Periodic Paralysis: The Mystery Unraveled,* which was the first book written exclusively about Periodic Paralysis, a mineral metabolic disorder. As we wrote in that book, it was "invented" or written out of necessity or an urgent need. The fact is there were no other up-to-date books written about Periodic Paralysis (PP) and information found on the Internet was scattered and sketchy at best. There was an urgent need to educate those with the different forms of Periodic Paralysis and their family members, as well as medical professionals, on all aspects of this condition. Our book did fill that need and covers all of the aspects of Periodic Paralysis. It is written in an easy to understand format. Part One contains an account of my medical issues from birth until the present. Part Two of the book covers every aspect of Periodic Paralysis. Part Three discusses the natural methods and technical information used to manage the symptoms by means of several "plans" with goals and objectives and instructions. Part Four deals with the emotional, psychological and social aspects related to living with Periodic Paralysis for the patient, caregiver and family.

The Periodic Paralysis Guide And Workbook: Be The Best You Can Be Naturally, also written in an easy to understand and user-friendly format, expands on Part Three and some of Part Four of our first book. This handbook has been designed as a tool to be used with the book or it may also stand-alone and may be used easily to achieve each goal and objective of the "plans" outlined in the book, using all natural and common sense methods.

The workbook begins with the basic facts and information about the various forms of Periodic Paralysis and the complications, both the more common ones and the more in-depth complications, which can develop and medical conditions, which can coexist with it. The second section includes information on educating oneself about Periodic Paralysis, learning to understand and describe paralytic episodes, identifying and eliminating all of the known triggers, relieving symptoms, monitoring vitals, securing a diagnosis, obtaining proper treatment, directing a medical team and more. Each plan is written in a series of simple goals and objectives and the methods to achieve success are explained and described. A set of tools such as charts, outlines and forms are included as well as a personal medical journal in the third section.

This guide is designed to also record, retain, save and store all of the important information about symptoms, triggers, treatment, medical information, family medical history, emergency information, treatment, vitals and more in one convenient place. Many charts and forms with explanation of how to use them may be copied or scanned. This handy workbook can easily accompany each visit to doctor appointments, the ER or hospital. It is a working tool, which can easily be added to as the needs or situation arises. It is a handy place to keep phone numbers and addresses of doctors, labs and hospitals. Medical professionals can easily copy the needed information for their records. It may be used for gaining a diagnosis or monitoring reactions to medications and more, but it is principally designed to assist individuals with Periodic Paralysis to be the best they can be, naturally in a user-friendly manner.

The information used in this workbook is compiled from our book, *living with Periodic Paralysis: The Mystery Unraveled;* our articles posted on our blog, *living with Periodic Paralysis: The Blog;* information shared and discussed on our Facebook *Periodic Paralysis Network Education, Support and Advocacy Discussion Group,* articles written on our *Periodic Paralysis Network Internet Website* and results retrieved from a set of surveys completed by the Periodic Paralysis Network, Inc.

The wealth of information in these sources was gleaned from a lifetime of experience and from over four years of experimentation, detailed research and tremendous study including, reading, analysis, exploration, investigation, trial and error, scrutiny, inquiry and more.

The references can be found in the following sources unless otherwise stated:

Knittle-Hunter, S and Hunter, C. 2013. Living with Periodic Paralysis: The Mystery Unraveled. Sequim, Washington. Periodic Paralysis Network.

Periodic Paralysis Network. (2014) Periodic Paralysis. Retrieved from:
http://www.periodicparalysisnetwork.com

Living With Periodic Paralysis: The Blog. (2014) Retrieved from:
http://livingwithperiodicparalysis.blogspot.com/

Another source of information mentioned and referred to in this book, is a set of surveys. The how and why of the information from the survey follows.

The Survey

Last year, not long after *living with Periodic Paralysis: The Mystery Unraveled* was published; I began working on this, our second book. However, shortly after that and within a few weeks of each other two members of our Periodic Paralysis Network Support Group traveled to see a Periodic Paralysis specialist in New York. One of them was clinically diagnosed and wanted to see a 'specialist' with the hope of better treatment options for her severe symptoms. Another member was seeking a diagnosis for her child.

The individual who was seeking a diagnosis for her child was immediately dismissed and treated very poorly after an EMG did not show any abnormalities. The odd thing about this is that the test can only diagnose a few forms of Periodic Paralysis and it is not necessary for the diagnosis of Periodic Paralysis. It is not conclusive either way, which means if it is negative it does not mean one does not have Periodic Paralysis and if it is positive it does not necessarily mean one has Periodic Paralysis. It is not always done correctly much of the time. To dismiss this little child and his family in such a manner based on this test was unconscionable.

The individual with a clinical diagnosis and seeking better treatment, was going to lose her insurance and wanted to get some help from the specialist before that happened because she was so ill and getting worse very quickly. Unbelievably, she was actually told by the same leading ATS specialist that she could not possibly have Periodic Paralysis due to the fact that her potassium levels were "TOO LOW". They actually drop

Getting Started

into the 1.0s!!! Low potassium levels are anything below 3.5. Her original clinical diagnosis was overturned, but ironically, she received confirmation of a genetic mutation for a form of Periodic Paralysis several months later for herself and other family members!!

Observing this happen to our members who are so ill and being treated so poorly by misinformed doctors in general and the "specialist" in particular was very concerning to me. Instead of continuing to write the second book about Periodic Paralysis, I immediately shifted gears and set out to create a set of criteria or a better and easier way to diagnose all forms of Periodic Paralysis clinically, based on symptoms and characteristics, rather than through genetic testing. This is because only about fifty percent of individuals with Periodic Paralysis have genetic mutations which have been located and the fact the most genetic testing for all forms of Periodic Paralysis is biased and too narrow in its scope, the chances of obtaining a genetic diagnosis are even further reduced.

I wrote a plan and created four comprehensive but informal surveys, covering the following areas: personal medical history, medical testing history, medication history, patient Periodic Paralysis symptoms and characteristics and family medical history. (The medical journal, other charts and forms in this book are actually designed from the survey.) We then utilized a reputable survey program to gather the information, professionally and anonymously, needed to create a new and better set of guidelines for better diagnosis of all forms of Periodic Paralysis based on an individuals symptoms and characteristics. We also hoped the information gathered, might help prove or at least throw suspicion on the existence of what we thought could be a new or overlooked form of Periodic Paralysis. We called this Periodic Paralysis Plus Ten Syndrome (PP+10S) in our first book.

Each survey took some time to complete and gather the information needed but by the time all four were concluded, we had 61 of our 100 members (at that time), who had participated. That provided us with enough information to began the work of studying the results and hopefully begin creating the new diagnosis project. As luck would have it, however, I ended up pushing myself too hard in order to get this all done and ended up having two small strokes. I had to put it all aside for a while as I recuperated. Unfortunately, I have never fully recovered but I have, however, begun to feel well enough to resume the project and complete our second book. The medical journal and other charts and forms in this book are actually designed from the survey.

The information and results gathered from our members were much as we expected and many things we suspected were confirmed. There were several surprises as well. I have decided to incorporate much of this information into this book, because some of the findings change the way we may now perceive or look at all forms of Periodic Paralysis and how to diagnose it. It is my hope that the medical professionals involved in Periodic Paralysis, may read this information and then search further into the findings, questions and speculations raised by the results. I hope also that they may study this information and use it to understand Periodic Paralysis and better be able to recognize and diagnose it.

Individualization

The Periodic Paralyses, mineral metabolic disorders, also known as ion channelopathies, are multifaceted and complicated. There are several known forms and many which have yet to be discovered. Therefore, recognizing, diagnosing and treating the symptoms of the various forms must be done on an individual basis.

Daily, on our PPNI Support Group, in private communication and even with my own family members, I am reminded that 'one size does not fit all' and 'what is good for the goose may not be good for the gander.' We are each different and the same treatments do not work for all of us. The drugs may be harmful to some of us. Some individuals may be able to eat sugar and others may not be able to eat it. Lidocaine may not pose a problem for some but may have serious side effects for others. Our episodes vary from person to person and even with ourselves. One time paralysis may last an hour the next time seven or eight hours. Some of us may be able to work and others are confined to a wheelchair. This book is created with this knowledge. Each person can totally individualize the goals and objectives for each selected plan to fit his or her unique needs.

In conclusion, every individual with any form of Periodic Paralysis; whether diagnosed genetically, clinically or still seeking a diagnosis; who reads this workbook, *The Periodic Paralysis Guide And Workbook: Be The Best You Can Be Naturally,* will be provided with up-to-date information regarding all aspects of Periodic Paralysis; will be provided with guidance on how to treat or improve the symptoms related to potassium shifting; will be provided with the tools to individualize each plan as needed, including but not limited to securing a diagnosis, finding a doctor and monitoring emergency care; will be provided with a few surprises and will be inspired to be the best he or she can be naturally and in a user friendly manner.

Now...Let's get started!!

One
Periodic Paralysis
THE BASIC FACTS

This workbook must begin with some basic facts about Periodic Paralysis including; what it is, the most common forms seen, how it is diagnosed, symptoms related to each type, triggers which may set it into motion, treatments for the symptoms and the expectations for the future. The basic facts are covered in this chapter to use as a quick reference. These will be expanded in more detail in the second chapter and throughout the following chapters.

Periodic Paralysis (PP) is a disease like no other. It is not a neuromuscular, mitochondrial or autoimmune disease nor is it a muscular dystrophy. It is in a category all its own and needs to be treated in non-conventional ways. Doctors need to keep an open mind and think 'outside of the box' when it comes to diagnosing and treating Periodic Paralysis.

The Basic Facts

Periodic Paralysis (PP) is an extremely rare, hereditary, mineral metabolic disorder characterized by episodes of muscular weakness or paralysis, a total lack of muscle tone without the loss of sensation while remaining conscious. It is passed from either the mother or the father to any of the children, male or female.

An Ion Channelopathy

Periodic Paralysis was one of the first ion channelopathies recognized. An ion channelopathy is a dysfunction of an ion channel, a microscopic tunnel in the cells of muscles called muscle fibers. Particles of potassium, sodium, chloride or calcium, which are electrically charged, known as ions, flow in and out of the cells. They regulate the contraction and relaxation of the muscle. A problem with the flow can cause paralysis. Channelopathies are considered metabolic disorders.

The Most Common Forms

Hypokalemic Periodic Paralysis (HypoPP)

Paralysis results from potassium moving from the blood into muscle cells in an abnormal way. It is associated with low levels of potassium in the blood (hypokalemia) during paralytic episodes.

Hyperkalemic Periodic Paralysis (HyperPP)

Paralysis results from problems with the way the body controls sodium and potassium levels in cells. It is associated with high levels of potassium in the blood (hyperkalemia) during paralytic episodes.

Andersen-Tawil Syndrome (ATS)

Paralysis results when the channel does not open properly; potassium cannot leave the cell. This disrupts the flow of potassium ions in skeletal and cardiac muscle. During paralytic episodes, ATS can be associated with low potassium, high potassium or shifts within the normal (normokalemia) ranges of potassium. An arrhythmia, long Qt interval heartbeat, is associated with ATS as well as certain characteristics, such as webbed or partially webbed toes, crooked little fingers and dental anomalies.

Normokalemic Periodic Paralysis (NormoPP)

Paralysis results when potassium shifts within in normal ranges. This can happen in any form of Periodic Paralysis; Hypokalemic Periodic Paralysis, Hyperkalemic Periodic Paralysis, Normokalemic Periodic Paralysis and Andersen-Tawil Syndrome. The paralysis may result from the shifting itself, rather than low or high potassium or it may occur due to the shifting of the potassium, which can happen very quickly and is undetectable in lab testing.

Paramyotonia Congenita (PMC)

The skeletal muscles can become stiff, tight, tense or contracted and weak due when the sodium channels close much too slowly and the sodium, potassium, chloride and water continue to flow into the muscles. It is actually considered to be a form of Hyperkalemic Periodic Paralysis, however, the symptoms can appear from shifting of potassium into low or high ranges or even if potassium shifts within normal levels.

Thyrotoxic Periodic Paralysis (TPP)

Intermittent paralysis results from low potassium due to an overactive thyroid or hyperthyroidism. It can occur spontaneously or can result from a genetic mutation. Unlike the other forms of Periodic Paralysis, TPP can be treated and cured by removing or treating the thyroid.

A large percentage of the above known types of Periodic Paralysis have identified genetic markers. This means they can be diagnosed by DNA testing.

Criteria For Making A Genetic Diagnosis

Hypokalemic Periodic Paralysis is caused by abnormalities in the SCN4A, KCNJ18 and CACNA1S genes.

Hyperkalemic Periodic Paralysis is caused by abnormalities in the SCN4A gene.

Andersen-Tawil Syndrome is caused by abnormalities in the KCNJ2 gene and the KCNJ5 gene.

Normokalemic Periodic Paralysis is caused by abnormalities in the SCN4A and CACNA1C genes.

Paramyotonia Congenita is caused by abnormalities in the SCN4A gene.

Thyrotoxic Periodic Paralysis is caused by abnormalities in the KCNE3 and KCNJ18 genes.

Criteria For Making A Clinical Diagnosis

Nearly one half of all cases of Periodic Paralysis do not have a known genetic cause, because the DNA mutations have not yet been discovered. A diagnosis can and should be made based on an individual's symptoms and characteristics. This is called being diagnosed "clinically." Those who are diagnosed clinically have symptoms and characteristics identical to others who have known genetic codes. For instance, one who is diagnosed with ATS clinically is said to have ATS Type 2 to differentiate from ATS Type 1. Clinical diagnosing is discussed in greater detail in Chapter Thirteen.

Symptoms

Although HypoPP, HyperPP, ATS, NormoPP and PMC are forms of periodic paralysis, the mechanism, which creates the muscle weakness and paralysis, is different as described above and the symptoms before and accompanying the paralysis vary. Symptoms can range from simple weakness to total body paralysis with life-threatening heart arrhythmias and tachycardia, breathing problems and choking. Death can occur in some rare cases. The episodes may last from a few minutes to several hours or many days. The speed with which the potassium shifts may cause symptoms to occur suddenly and without warning or there may be a gradual progression into the weakness or paralysis.

Abortive attacks may also affect some individuals. Occasionally, the common symptoms may begin but the full attack or paralysis may not occur. The person is left with extreme weakness and other symptoms such as extreme fatigue. This may last for hours, days, weeks or even months. In some cases the abortive attack is totally debilitating and actually worse than the episodes of paralysis. Symptoms are discussed further in Chapters Eight and Eleven.

Triggers

The periodic muscle weakness or paralysis is triggered by a wide variety of activities such as exercise or sleep; foods such as carbohydrates or meat; conditions such as heat or cold; medications such as antibiotics or muscle relaxers; compounds such as caffeine or salt or simply resting after exercise. Many of the triggers are the same for most people but some of the triggers can be unique to each person or the type of Periodic Paralysis. Triggers are discussed in greater detail in Chapters Ten and Eleven.

Treatment

Many of the individuals with Hypokalemic Periodic Paralysis are able to control the symptoms and paralytic attacks with one or two forms of potassium and avoiding the things that trigger them. Individuals with Hyperkalemic Periodic Paralysis symptoms and paralytic attacks can control their symptoms and paralytic attacks with a diet high in carbohydrates and sugar and by avoiding the triggers.

Normokalemic Periodic Paralysis should not be treated with potassium because the potassium levels remain in the normal ranges and raising the potassium levels may cause hyperkalemia. Avoiding triggers is necessary.

Controlling the symptoms and paralytic attacks in people with Andersen-Tawil Syndrome is much more difficult. This is due to the fact that these individuals suffer from paralysis due to potassium levels that can be low, high or in normal ranges. Taking potassium may make the symptoms worse. Also individuals with ATS are usually unable to take any forms of medication. Managing the heart issues by surgery is also a problem because anesthesia can trigger paralysis and deadly arrythmia. For these individuals, natural methods are the best way to manage the symptoms.

When treating the symptoms of Paramyotonia Congenita, treating it like Hyperkalemic Periodic Paralysis is the most common method however, because PMC may accompany any form of Periodic Paralysis, episodes may be precipitated by low or high potassium, or even shifting within normal ranges so monitoring the levels of potassium is important and treatment should be based on the potassium levels and the symptoms accompanying the episodes. Treatments are discussed in more detail in Chapter Eleven.

More in-depth information about the various forms of Periodic Paralysis is found in the following chapter and throughout this book and can also be found in *living with Periodic Paralysis: The Mystery Unraveled* and in the PPNI Blog.

Two
The Periodic Paralyses
MORE DETAIL

Although all known as Periodic Paralysis, or the Periodic Paralyses, each form is very different in how and why it presents, what things trigger the symptoms and how to treat and manage them. More in-depth detail and information for all forms of Periodic Paralysis is discussed in this chapter.

Hypokalemic Periodic Paralysis

Hypokalemic Periodic Paralysis, also known as Westphall Disease, is the most common form of Periodic Paralysis accounting for about 70% of all cases. If an individual has Hypokalemic Periodic Paralysis he or she become partially or fully paralyzed intermittently. As already stated, the paralysis results from potassium moving from the blood into muscle cells in an abnormal way. It is associated with low levels of potassium (hypokalemia) during paralytic episodes.

When potassium shifts into lower ranges in normal individuals, it is called hypokalemia. Low potassium levels in the blood will occur for anyone and a myriad of symptoms may be experienced and can be dangerous, even deadly. If an individual has Hypokalemic Periodic Paralysis and potassium shifts into lower ranges, he or she can and will experience a combination of the same myriad of symptoms as well as paralysis and can be equally as dangerous and deadly.

When potassium levels are low, which is usually between 2.5 to 3.5 mEq/L, the following symptoms can occur: tiredness, pain in the muscles, cramping, upset stomach, constipation, lightheadedness, depression, mood swings.

Potassium levels below 2.5 mEq/L affect many functions of the body including the muscles, digestion, kidneys, electrolyte balance, the liver and the heart.

Muscles: fatigue, pain in the joints, muscle weakness, muscle weakness after exercise, muscle stiffness, muscle aches, muscle cramps, muscle contractions, muscle spasms, muscle tenderness, pins and needles sensation, eyelid myotonia (cannot open eyelid after opening and then closing them).

Digestion: Upset stomach, loss of appetite, vomiting, constipation, diarrhea, bloating of the stomach and full feeling in the stomach, blockage in the intestines called paralytic ileus.

Heart: Anxiousness, irregular and rapid heartbeat, angina, prominent U waves, inverted or flattened T waves, ST depression, elongated PR interval.

Kidneys: Severe thirst, increased urination, difficulty breathing, too slow or shallow breathing, lack of oxygen in the blood, sweating, increased blood pressure, metabolic acidosis.

Liver: The brain function becomes affected: Irritability, decrease in concentration, lack of clear thinking, confusion, slurring of speech, seizures.

Paralysis: Episodic muscle weakness, episodic partial paralysis, episodic total paralysis episodic flaccid paralysis (limp muscles, without tone).

Laboratory blood changes: Increased number of neutrophils in blood, increased number of white blood cells in the blood, reduced number of eosinophils in blood, increased number of lymphocytes in blood, low blood sodium, low blood potassium, elevated Serum CPK (creatine).

Laboratory urine changes: Excess protein in urine, excess sugar in the urine, excessive acetone in urine, and presence of renal casts in urine.

An individual with Periodic Paralysis may have his or her own individual levels of potassium at which symptoms or paralysis occurs. What may be normal ranges for someone may be high for another. Using a potassium reader to discover one's high, normal and low ranges is suggested, for better treatment.

Factors, which can trigger attacks, are: Excessive carbohydrates, alcoholic beverages, sodium/salt, viruses, certain medications, epinephrine, cold, anesthesia, excitement/fear, exercise, and rest or sleep (all phases).

Attacks of paralysis may be reduced by: Eating high potassium foods, staying warm, staying well rested, staying hydrated, avoiding drugs that decrease potassium levels, avoiding known triggers such as stress, exercise, carbohydrates, and salt.

Some off-label drugs, which can be effective for treating the symptoms, are available for some individuals with Hypokalemic Periodic Paralysis but they should be used with extreme caution due to serious side effects.

Hyperkalemic Periodic Paralysis

Hyperkalemic Periodic Paralysis, also known as Gamstorp Disease, accounts for about 15 to 20% of all forms of Periodic Paralysis. If an individual has Hyperkalemic Periodic Paralysis he or she becomes partially or fully paralyzed intermittently based on the way the body controls sodium and potassium levels in the cells. It is associated with high levels of potassium (hyperkalemia) during paralytic episodes.

When potassium shifts into higher ranges in normal individuals, it is called hyperkalemia. High potassium levels in the blood will occur for anyone and a myriad of symptoms may be experienced and can be dangerous, even deadly. If an individual has Hyperkalemic Periodic Paralysis and potassium shifts into higher ranges, he or she can and will experience a combination of the same myriad of symptoms as well as paralysis and can be equally as dangerous and deadly.

The Periodic Paralyses

When potassium levels are at a slightly elevated level there may be no symptoms. At a moderately higher level, which is usually between 5.5 and 6.5 mEq/L, there may be some symptoms involving muscles, digestion, kidneys, electrolyte balance, the liver and the heart.

Potassium levels above 6.5 mEq/L are very serious and usually require medical attention.

Muscles: Fatigue, weakness, pins and needles, tingling or numbness in the extremities, muscle contraction, muscle rigidity, muscle cramps, muscles stiffness, muscle twitching, muscle cramping, reduced reflexes, muscle contraction involving tongue, tightness in legs, strange feeling in legs.

Digestion: Discomfort, nausea, vomiting, stomach cramps, diarrhea, vomiting.
Heart: Palpitations, chest pain, irregular heartbeat, slow heartbeat, weak pulse, absent pulse, heart stoppage, small P waves, tall T waves, QRS abnormality, P wave abnormality, QT lengthening, fast heartbeat.

Kidneys: Breathing problems, wheezing, shortness of breath, fast breathing, feeling hot, low blood pressure.

Liver: The brain function becomes affected: Irritability, sleepiness, confusion, seizures, and loss of consciousness.

Paralysis: Episodic muscle weakness, episodic partial paralysis, episodic total paralysis.
Laboratory blood changes: Elevated blood potassium, serum sodium level elevated, Serum CPK (creatine).

Laboratory urine changes: Elevated urine pH level.

An individual with Periodic Paralysis may have his or her own individual levels of potassium at which symptoms or paralysis occurs. What may be normal ranges for someone may be high for another. Using a potassium reader to discover one's high, normal and low ranges is suggested, for better treatment.

Factors which can trigger attacks include rest after exercise, potassium-rich foods, stress, fatigue, weather changes, certain pollutants (especially cigarette smoke), periods of fasting, cold temperatures, certain anesthetics, depolarizing muscle relaxants, other medications which increase potassium levels, alcohol and heavy exercise.

Attacks may be reduced by: Avoiding high potassium foods, drugs known to increase potassium level and fasting. Also it is important to stay warm, engage in mild regular exercise if possible eat a diet high in carbohydrates and avoid known triggers.

Off-label drugs, which can be effective for treating the symptoms, are available for some individuals with Hyperkalemic Periodic Paralysis but they should be used with extreme caution due to serious side effects.

The Periodic Paralysis Guide And Workbook

Andersen-Tawil Syndrome

Andersen-Tawil Syndrome, also known as Long QT Syndrome 7, is the most rare and the most serious form and accounts for about 10% of all cases of Periodic Paralysis. It is characterized by three particular components: periods of paralysis from high, low or normal potassium levels, distinctive crania-facial and skeletal characteristics and long QT interval heartbeat with a predisposition toward life-threatening ventricular arrhythmia. However, affected individuals may express only one or two of the three components and they may be very subtle. Other characteristics and abnormalities are also associated with Andersen-Tawil Syndrome.

These physical abnormalities and characteristics associated with Andersen-Tawil Syndrome are as follows:

Characteristics and Features:
(May be very subtle, partial or seen in 'unaffected' family members)
Skeletal:
- Delayed bone age (slowed degree of maturation of child's bones)
- Short stature
- Scoliosis (curved spine)

Dental:
- Hypodontia (born with missing teeth)
- Persistent primary dentition (still have some baby teeth)

Hands and Feet:
- Brachydactyly (unusually short fingers)
- Brachydactyly type D (clubbed thumbs) (characterized by a slightly shorter thumb that is round in section and larger at the end)
- Clinodactyly (inward curvature/ 5th fingers)
- Syndactyly (webbing between fingers or between 2nd and 3rd toes)

Face:
- Short palpebral fissures (short opening for the eyes between the eyelids)
- Ocular hypertelorism (widely spaced eyes);
- Microcephaly (abnormal smallness of the head)
- Broad nasal root (wide space between the inner corners of eyes)
- Broad forehead (increased distance between the two sides of the forehead or top to bottom of forehead)
- Malar hypolasia (small cheek bones)
- Micrognathia (short jaw)
- Prognathism (protruding jaw)
- Ptosis (an abnormally low position (drooping) of the upper eyelid)
- Low set ears

Mouth
- Small mandible (lower jaw in which the lower teeth reside and chin)
- Hypoplasia of maxilla (small upper jaw)
- Cleft palate (a congenital fissure in the roof of the mouth)
- High arched palate (roof of the mouth is high)

Joints
- Joint laxity (looseness of the muscles and soft tissue surrounding a joint

Heart
- ❖ Ventricular arrhythmia
- ❖ Abnormal heart rhythm
- ❖ Long QT syndrome (increased time needed for heart to recharge after each heartbeat)
- ❖ Irregular heartbeat
- ❖ Fainting caused by irregular heartbeat

Executive Functioning (EF) Disorder can accompany ATS

There are three primary layers of executive functions:
- ❖ Self-regulation
- ❖ Organization
- ❖ High order reasoning skills

It is associated with many disabilities:
- ❖ Attention Deficit Hyperactivity Disorder (AD/HD)
- ❖ Learning Disabilities (LD)
- ❖ Tourette Syndrome (TS)
- ❖ Obsessive Compulsive Disorder (OCD)
- ❖ Autism
- ❖ Depression

At this time, there are two recognized types of Andersen-Tawil syndrome, Type 1 and Type 2, which are distinguished only by their genetic causes. One has a known genetic mutation and the other, though the symptoms and characteristics are exactly the same, has no known genetic mutation, which has been discovered.

In most of the textbook or journal articles, Andersen-Tawil Syndrome is described as being so rare that only one hundred cases have been diagnosed worldwide. This is incorrect. In a part of France alone, over seventy-two cases exist in nine surveyed hospitals. One hundred cases of ATS is a gross underestimation. Far more cases exist in varying forms. It is not recognized, it is misdiagnosed and it is under diagnosed.

Factors that can trigger attacks include any of the triggers for Hypokalemic Periodic Paralysis and for Hyperkalemic Periodic Paralysis.

For Individuals with Andersen-Tawil Syndrome, avoiding episodes of paralysis is extremely important and can be done by avoiding all of the known triggers. Anesthesia and off-label drugs, which can be effective for treating the symptoms of the other forms of Periodic Paralysis, should be avoided as well as any other drugs or medications, especially those that cause long QT heartbeats.

Normokalemic Periodic Paralysis

Normokalemic Periodic Paralysis is a form of Periodic Paralysis in which the potassium does not shift out of normal ranges, however an individual becomes partially or fully paralyzed intermittently. The paralysis results from the actual shifting of the potassium. This may happen in any form of Periodic Paralysis and there are also specific genetic mutations responsible for this. This is discussed further and in great detail in Chapter Five.

Paramyotonia Congenita

Paramyotonia Congenita, also known as Von Eulenberg's Disease, is an important form or Periodic Paralysis. It affects the muscles used in movement. Caused by certain triggers, the sodium channels close much too slowly and the sodium, potassium, chloride and water continue to flow into the muscles. The skeletal muscles can become stiff, tight, tense or contracted and weak. In the same family, some members may have mild forms and others may have more extreme cases. It is actually considered to be a form of Hyperkalemic Periodic Paralysis, however, the symptoms can appear from shifting of potassium into low or high ranges or even if potassium shifts within normal levels. Symptoms can begin shortly after birth or during childhood or at anytime in early adulthood.

Myotonia is the prolonged or lengthy contraction, tensing or lack of relaxation of a muscle or group of skeletal muscles, which is relieved by exercise. For those with Paramyotonia Congenita, the contractions or tightness are not relieved by exercise. The symptoms or muscle tightness are brought on by triggers such as exercise or exertion, repeated movement and cold. It is also known that episodes are common in the early morning so sleeping in, in the morning, may cause episodes. Hands, face and eyelids are often seen affected. It can be seen as simply a hand cramp while writing or the inability to let go of something being held in the hand like a door knob or the affects can be as significant as total body paralysis with contracted and tight muscles. The episodes can last for minutes, hours or days. There may also be intermittent flaccid paralysis as in the other types of Periodic Paralysis in which there is no muscle tone and the muscles are totally loose and slack. Because breathing muscles may be affected, shortness of breath may accompany episodes. Episodes may be mild or very severe and pain may be experienced even after the episode has ended. Individuals with PMC may appear to be stiff or look tense, even when not in an episode.

There is some difference of opinion as to whether PMC is a progressive condition, but more recent analysis and study of patients with it, indicates that some individuals may have some progressive and permanent muscle weakness.

Avoiding known triggers is the best treatment. Some individuals respond well to the common medications used for Periodic Paralysis, but the side effects can be worse than the symptoms. Because extremes of any type can cause episodes, moderation of everything and anything is important. A pH balanced diet can also be helpful because a high pH can cause symptoms and episodes to be eliminated or shortened. Also, due to the fact that low or high potassium, or even shifting within normal ranges may precipitate episodes, the levels of potassium must be evaluated individually for each person.

Individuals with Paramyotonia Congenita/Hyperkalemic Periodic Paralysis are at great risk for Malingnant Hyperthermia, severe reactions to general anesthesia. Extreme care must be used if surgery is needed.

Thyrotoxic Periodic Paralysis

Thyrotoxic Periodic Paralysis, also known as Thyrotoxic Hypokalemic Periodic Paralysis, is a form of Periodic Paralysis related to thyroid dysfunction that creates high thyroid hormone. If an individual has Thyrotoxic Periodic Paralysis he or she becomes partially or fully paralyzed intermittently based on low potassium levels. The symptoms are the same as if an individual has Hypokalemic Periodic Paralysis.

Although some forms can occur without a known cause, it is now known that some types are caused by genetic mutation. Symptoms are treated just as Hypokalemic Periodic Paralysis is treated, but unlike the other forms of Periodic Paralysis, Thyrotoxic Periodic Paralysis can be treated and cured by treating the thyroid dysfunction or by removing it.

Survey Results For Forms Of Period Paralysis

Our survey indicated that 72% of our members were diagnosed. Twenty-two percent were genetically diagnosed and 50% were diagnosed clinically. Of those members diagnosed, 60% had Hypokalemic Periodic Paralysis, 3% had Hyperkalemic Periodic Paralysis and 8% had Andersen-Tawil Syndrome. Though none were diagnosed with Normokalemic Periodic Paralysis, 58% had episodes within normal ranges. None were diagnosed with Thyrotoxic Periodic Paralysis or Paramyotonia Congenita, though some had symptoms to suggest it.

http://livingwithperiodicparalysis.blogspot.com/2014/01/what-is-hypokalemic-periodic-paralysis.html
http://livingwithperiodicparalysis.blogspot.com/2013/12/what-is-hyperkalemic-periodic-paralysis.html
http://livingwithperiodicparalysis.blogspot.com/2013/12/what-is-andersen-tawil-syndrome.html
http://livingwithperiodicparalysis.blogspot.com/2014/02/what-is-normokalemic-periodic-paralysis.html
http://livingwithperiodicparalysis.blogspot.com/2014/05/paramyotonia-congenita-another-form-of.html

Three
An Ion Channelopathy
A MINERAL METABOLIC DISORDER

Periodic Paralysis is an ion channelopathy. Ion channelopathies are considered a class four metabolic disorder, therefore, Periodic Paralysis is a fourth class mineral metabolic disorder. An ion channelopathy is a dysfunction of an ion channel. Ion channelopathies were first recognized in 1971 and Andersen-Tawil Syndrome was the first to be discovered.

Ion channels are like a microscopic tunnel in the cells of muscles. The tunnels are called muscle fibers. Ions, which are molecules or atoms, flow in and out of the muscle cells through membranes or gates. Each of the gates is shaped exactly for the correct ion or molecule to enter. The ions are made up of what we call minerals, electrolytes or proteins. Some of the common ions are potassium, sodium, magnesium, chloride and calcium. They are electrically charged and each has its own size or shape, so to speak. If the gates or membranes are faulty in size or shape, an inefficient or improper flow through the membranes can and does cause muscle weakness and paralysis because they regulate contraction and relaxation of the muscle.

Disorders of metabolism are usually inherited and are involved in chemical and physical processing, which use and make energy in the body. These processes include: breathing, circulation of blood, food and nutrient digestion, elimination of waste through bowel and bladder and temperature regulation.

Unfortunately, ion channelopathies are not usually categorized nor listed in medical writing or studies as metabolic disorders. This poses a problem for recognition, diagnosis and treatment by physicians and other medical professionals. Periodic Paralysis, which is a channelopathy, is often referred to as a neuromuscular disease (affecting muscles and/or nerves also known as myoneural), a muscular dystrophy (wasting of muscle and eventual early death), or a disease of the nervous system (nothing to do with the nervous system), but none of these is correct. Periodic Paralysis is a metabolic disorder, a condition which is based in the faulty cellular level of how energy is produced in our bodies.

To clarify, even further, Periodic Paralysis is a channelopathy which is a mineral metabolic disorder. Metabolism disorders involving minerals are conditions in which there is either not enough or an overabundance of minerals in an individual's blood. Minerals have many functions in metabolism and the functions of the human body. They are important in bone and muscle building and growth. Organs, cells and tissues need minerals in order to function properly. So, a dysfunction of minerals in the body affects many processes and functions. Potassium, the main mineral involved in Periodic Paralysis, is involved in making proteins from the amino acids and plays a role in carbohydrate metabolism, so a dysfunction involving it, can affect more than just muscles.

The doctors most often seen for this condition are almost always neurologists. This is a problem when seeking a diagnosis and treatment because Periodic Paralysis is not a neuromuscular disease and although it affects the muscles, the treatments involved should not be those used for neuromuscular diseases. Some confusion about this may come from the fact that the Muscular Dystrophy Association (MDA) lists it as one of the diseases they research and treat. They are known for diagnosing and treating muscle wasting diseases. Periodic Paralysis is not a muscle wasting disease though on rare occasion there can be muscle wasting.

The probable reason most individuals with Periodic Paralysis end up with a neurologist, or a number of them, is because the symptoms look like a neurological disease. Neurologists, however, can be good for ruling out a neuromuscular disease, but at the point it is ruled out, then an individual should be referred to a doctor specializing in metabolic disorders. However, this is the point when conversion disorder or hypochondria becomes the diagnosis instead.

This clarification in the medical field could help us to get better treatment and quicker diagnoses, by seeing the correct physicians. That being said, an endocrinologist should be the correct doctor to see. However, many of them are not aware of Periodic Paralysis. How to find a doctor and get a diagnosis are discussed later in this book.

http://livingwithperiodicparalysis.blogspot.com/2014/01/what-is-ion-channelopathy.html

Four
Possible Complications
THE MOST COMMON

There is no doubt that many complications are associated with Periodic Paralysis, especially when the condition has been misdiagnosed and mistreated over many years. The following are some of the more common complications found in many individuals with all forms of Periodic Paralysis.

Progressive Permanent Muscle Weakness (PMW)

Muscle weakness is a decrease in the strength of muscle and the need for extra effort in order to move the affected muscles in the body. It can involve the function and movement of one or more muscle groups. It can be very mild for some and totally debilitating for others. It can be the inability to do specific things like walking up stairs or reaching above one's head. Muscle weakness is the result of a number of diseases of the skeletal muscles. These include the muscle dystrophies, the inflammatory muscle diseases, the neuromuscular diseases and the muscle myopathy diseases. The cause of the muscle weakness will determine which muscle or muscle groups will be affected. A generalized muscle weakness is one that involves the entire body.

In Periodic Paralysis, which is a mineral metabolic myopathy, also known as an inherited myopathy, there is generalized weakness, because the muscles of the entire body are involved. There is no loss of sensation or feeling, however. The weakness is usually most noticeable in what are called the proximal muscles, those closest to the trunk, and the largest of the muscle groups. The weakness is equal on both sides of the body. And, although the weakness and paralysis are intermittent and have a beginning and an end in most cases, for some the weakness becomes chronic, or occurring over a long span of time or it returns often. The chronic weakness can become slowly progressive and fixed or permanent. Once it becomes chronic it can cause muscle wasting and fat or lipid can replace the muscle as we have seen in a previous chapter. At the point the muscle weakness becomes permanent, it will not go away and at this point it is progressive meaning it will steadily continue to worsen.

Symptoms

The symptoms of progressive muscle weakness begin with general muscle weakness. The weakness gradually increases as endurance decreases and muscle wasting can be seen. The progressing weakness can cause an imbalance of the joints causing restricted movement. This in turn can lead to deformities as well as stiffness. This begins in the thighs, shoulders and upper arms and the muscles closest to the trunk. Then as it advances it spreads to the muscles of the feet and hands.

In Periodic Paralysis the large muscle groups are obviously affected, those attached to bone and also the muscles for breathing, talking and eating, the muscles of the throat and the eyes and of course, the heart being a muscle, it can be affected also. This means that as it progresses some of the functions of the body that can be affected are, but not limited to, standing, walking (gait, coordination and reflexes), sitting, rising from a chair, using arms (reaching above the head), and hands (writing, typing and feeding oneself), talking, eating, chewing, swallowing, digestion, elimination (bladder and bowels), breathing, vision and heart rate and rhythm. Once it begins to affect the muscles of the chest, the breathing or respiratory muscles, Periodic Paralysis becomes terminal.

My own symptoms of muscle weakness came on very gradually as would be expected, though as a child I experienced weakness for as long as I can remember. I first noticed a problem with walking up inclines and then stairs.

Diagnosing

Tests can be performed to confirm the muscle wasting. Of course a physical examination would be first, then laboratory studies including a study of muscle enzymes would be in order, as well as, electromyography (study of electrical activity of muscles), which can confirm the myopathy and types of radiology (MRI's, x-rays) may be used. The most invasive of the tests is a muscle biopsy. A surgical procedure, using anesthesia, is performed to remove a piece of muscle to study in a laboratory.

If a muscle biopsy is performed few abnormalities will appear for an individual with Periodic Paralysis unless permanent damage to the muscles has occurred. Changes in size and shape of muscle fibers may be found as well as lipids. There may also be changes in the vacuoles, an increase in fibers with internal nuclei and the formation of excess connective tissue.

Care should be given if a muscle biopsy is to be used. Lidocaine is a serious trigger for paralysis and arrhythmias in Periodic Paralysis. I had a muscle biopsy performed, before my diagnosis, to rule out mitochondrial disease. I had some complications with the lidocaine. The test results did indicate, however, the existence of mild muscle myopathy. It was discovered that I had changes in size and shape of some muscle fibers. Also noted was the existence of fatty tissue.

Treatment for Progressive Muscle Weakness

If an individual has Periodic Paralysis we know there is no cure or treatment for permanent progressive muscle weakness. There is no way to strengthen the muscles involved in breathing once they are permanently weakened. Although the literature regarding permanent muscle weakness indicates that physical therapy can be helpful for all individuals with muscle weakness, this is not true for those with Periodic Paralysis. It can actually be more harmful to exercise due to exercise intolerance.

http://livingwithperiodicparalysis.blogspot.com/2014/01/permanent-muscle-weakness-in-periodic.html
http://livingwithperiodicparalysis.blogspot.com/2014/01/permanent-muscle-weakness-in-periodic_12.html

Exercise Intolerance

We know that there are two types of involvement of muscles in individuals with Periodic Paralysis. There are attacks of paralysis of the muscles, which are intermittent, and there is a myopathy or a progressive, permanent muscle weakness, which can occur. Some individuals experience one or the other and some experience both conditions, though it is

Possible Complications

less common to have both, and it is very rare to have only the progressive, permanent muscle weakness. If an individual develops the progressive, permanent form of periodic paralysis, it begins as exercise intolerance, usually in the legs and feet, which progressively spreads to the rest of the muscles in the body.

In exercise intolerance the individual is not able to do physical exercise or exertion that would be expected from someone of his or her age and overall health level nor for the amount of time expected. He or she lacks stamina. The individual may also experience extreme pain and fatigue after exercising or exertion and other symptoms such as a feeling of heaviness in the muscle groups. Exercise intolerance is a symptom rather than a condition or disease. It is a common symptom found in several diseases including metabolic disorders. Periodic Paralysis is a mineral metabolic myopathy.

Food and oxygen are normally converted into energy and delivered to the muscles but this cycle is disrupted in individuals with exercise intolerance. The muscles are unable to use the nutrients and oxygen and therefore, enough energy may not be generated to the muscles and he or she is left with little or no energy. The degrees of low energy can be mild or extreme and the symptoms may occur during exercise or exertion or they can occur later, even the next day.

Symptoms

Symptoms of exercise intolerance include: fatigue, muscle cramps, insufficient heart rate, depression, changes in blood pressure and cyanosis. Fatigue may show within minutes of beginning to exercise with shortness of breath or dizziness. This is a sign that sufficient oxygen is not being processed. For individuals with severe exercise intolerance this can happen after doing simple tasks such as eating, sitting up in a chair or writing. Muscle cramping and stiffness also will appear within a few minutes of beginning to exercise. This can linger for days after the exercising. There may also be a delayed reaction of hours and the pain may begin while one is sleeping causing one to awaken. The heart rate does not increase enough to meet the needs of the muscles during the activity. Depression is often seen in individuals with exercise intolerance. Not being able to do the things a person wants to do or should be able to do can create anxiety, irritability, bewilderment and hopelessness leading to depression. Standing up or walking across a room may be all that is necessary for an individual's blood pressure to rise significantly. Cyanosis is a serious condition that indicates there is not enough oxygen in the blood. The individual may appear to look blue in the face and hands and needs immediate medical attention.

Exercise intolerance can be seen in the small muscle groups as well as the large muscle groups. Writing or other fine motor skills can be affected causing cramping, fatigue and spasms. Tachycardia (fast heart beats) can occur from increased breathing rate during exercise or exertion and this rapid breathing can increases from fatigue of the diaphragm and chest wall. Vision may become blurry due to fatigue of the eye muscles. The oral muscles, those involving the mouth, may be affected making speech difficult and making chewing of harder or tougher foods a problem.

Diagnosing

Diagnosis would be based on the symptoms above and the diagnosis of the root cause, which in this case is Periodic Paralysis.

Treatment

For most individuals with Periodic Paralysis who have exercise intolerance, it is best to avoid physical activity and exertion because it can lead to muscle cell damage (muscle wasting), exhaustion and a condition called lactic acidosis, a form of metabolic acidosis (also discussed in this book). It also can be a trigger for attacks of paralysis.

http://livingwithperiodicparalysis.blogspot.com/2014/07/exercise-intolerance.html

Heart Issues

Abnormal heart rhythms are serious and life-threatening complications for individuals with Periodic Paralysis. Each of the three forms, Hypokalemic Periodic Paralysis, Hyperkalemic Periodic Paralysis and Anderson-Tawil Syndrome, has a specific pattern of irregular heartbeats, which makes it easy to identify on an electrical study of the heart called an electrocardiogram (EKG). It is not necessary to explain or understand each irregular heartbeat or pattern. They are however, referenced in the following sections for recognition and for diagnosis by physicians and patients.

Hypokalemic Periodic Paralysis

When an individual with Periodic Paralysis begins to experience a decrease in potassium, there is a decrease in the "T" wave. The next step is an "ST- segment depression" and then the "T" waves become inverted or "flip". At the same time the "PR" interval becomes prolonged and the "P" wave enlarges. A "U" wave appears after the "T" wave and can be seen on the mid-precordial leads. When the "U" wave becomes larger than the "T" wave develops on the EKG, the potassium level in less than 3 (<3). As the potassium levels decrease further, the "T' and "U" wave combine into a prominent "U" wave on the EKG. This makes the "T" waves visible.

At this point, in severe hypokalemia, a person might also develop ventricular tachycardia (fast heart beat) and/or ventricular fibrillation. The fibers of the ventricle of the heart contract in an uncontrolled and random manner. When this happens, without immediate medical help, the individual will die because the heart can stop beating suddenly and unexpectedly from cardiac arrest. Occasionally atrioventricular block, which is a sudden pause or bradycardia that is a slow heartbeat (under 60 beats per minute) can occur. So, in episodes of hypokalemia in individuals with Periodic Paralysis, there may be either a fast heartbeat or a slow heartbeat along with the specific arrhythmia.

Hyperkalemic Periodic Paralysis

If an individual has mild to moderately high potassium levels in his or her blood, "P" wave becomes smaller in size and a peaked "T" wave develops on an electrocardiogram (EKG). In more dangerous higher levels of potassium it affects the electrical conduction of the heart in the sinoatrial (SA) of the heart. The SA is the "pacemaker" of the heart and responsible for the contraction of a heart beat.

On an EKG the "P" wave disappears and the ventricular contraction lengthens. This appears on an EKG as a "QRS complex". The overall pumping of the heart decreases to below 60 beats per minute and this is called bradycardia. The pulse becomes weak and heart block may occur. There may also be an increase in the heart rate called ventricular tachycardia. Arrhythmias in the form of ventricular fibrillation may also occur. So, in episodes of hyperkalemia in individuals with Periodic Paralysis, there may be either a fast heartbeat or a slow heartbeat along with the specific arrhythmia.

Andersen-Tawil Syndrome:

In an individual with Andersen-Tawil Syndrome, the heart complications are very distinctive, extremely serious and some of the arrhythmias are life threatening. They can include prominent two-phased "U" waves, down sloped terminal "T" waves which are prolonged, wide "TU" waves, premature ventricular complexes (PVCs), ventricular arrhythmias, including ventricular tachycardia, ventricular tachycardia which is bidirectional (BVT), supraventricular tachycardia, ventricular fibrillation, long QT interval heart beat (a ventricular tachycardia) and torsades de pointes.

He or she may have no symptoms although they are experiencing arrhythmias, or they may have minor symptoms despite experiencing a serious number of arrhythmias and tachycardia or they may be very symptomatic. Regardless of the symptoms, a person is at high-risk for sudden death from an arrhythmia, namely the long QT heartbeat (LQT), the torsades de pointes and the ventricular fibrillation.

The changes, which are most common and affect the heart most often in Andersen-Tawil Syndrome, are the ventricular arrhythmias. This is a disruption in the lower chambers of the heart. In the long QT heart beat the heart muscle takes longer than normal between beats to recharge. When this condition is not treated it leads to uncomfortable feelings, syncope, (fainting) or cardiac arrest. The long QT interval heartbeat is one of the distinguishing features used to identify and diagnose Andersen-Tawil Syndrome.

There may be no actual, underlying cardiac disease in individuals with Andersen-Tawil Syndrome, but rather they are born with the predisposition to develop, under certain circumstances (triggers), the ventricular tachycardia and arrhythmias identified here. However, cardiomyopathy, a disease of the heart muscle, often develops in persons with Anderson-Tawil Syndrome. The heart becomes thickened and/or enlarged and weakens. This leads to heart failure.

Diagnosing

Diagnosing Hypokalemic Periodic Paralysis, Hyperkalemic Periodic Paralysis or Andersen-Tawil Syndrome, based on the patterns on an EKG or a twenty-four hour Holter Monitor, should be very straightforward based on the previous outlined information, when combined with the other symptoms unique to Periodic Paralysis, especially the intermittent paralysis or muscle weakening occurring as the EKG is being recorded. However, in many cases, this is not being used as part of the diagnosis and is often overlooked, misread or ignored.

The Need for Oxygen

Symptoms

The potassium shifting and depletion that occurs in Periodic Paralysis can affect all the muscles of the body including the heart muscle and the respiratory (breathing) muscles. The muscles can become permanently weakened and this includes the heart and breathing muscles. This weakness of the heart muscle and breathing muscles can be fatal in Periodic Paralysis. The diaphragm is the primary breathing muscle. The intercostal muscles are secondary breathing muscles. Breathing involves all the muscles from mouth to lower abdomen. Paralysis of the diaphragm can cause respiratory arrest or the sudden stoppage of breathing.

If the organs are deprived of oxygen, the heart and the rest of the body are working harder to stay alive. This can cause an individual with PP to develop hypoventilation. This is a condition in which one is barely breathing due to weak breathing muscles which prompts him or her to breath less and less over time. Eventually one will get accustomed to getting by on less oxygen while excess carbon dioxide is stored in his muscles and organs. This can cause long-term problems including damage to most of the organs and muscles in the body, but the heart and brain are particularly vulnerable. Oxygen therapy may be necessary at this point.

Based on the above information, it is important to understand that when someone with Periodic Paralysis begins to hyperventilate during an episode with tachycardia, this is due to the body trying to compensate by expelling the excess carbon dioxide. This is a good thing, though he or she may be trying to stop the process, because it may be scary. A caregiver should allow the person to hyperventilate without resorting to such things as using a paper bag.

And so, if an individual, who may or not be on oxygen therapy, begins to have difficulty breathing during an episode of partial or total paralysis or at any time; he or she may get some relief if they breathe in through their nose and breathe out as hard as they can through the mouth to expel the carbon dioxide. It is good to do this until the breathing becomes easier and oxygen levels rise. The use of a portable finger oximeter is helpful in self-monitoring oxygen levels at home.

One can develop a serious condition of metabolic acidosis if the carbon dioxide levels are allowed to rise and remain in the body. Metabolic acidosis affects the cardiovascular and respiratory systems. It can cause potassium to shift out of the cells creating hyperkalemia. Hyperkalemia, which is high levels of potassium, and metabolic acidosis, a pH imbalance in which the body has accumulated too much acid and does not have enough bicarbonate to effectively neutralize the effects of the acid, can be life threatening.

Some individuals with Periodic Paralysis and Andersen-Tawil Syndrome must be careful with exercise if they begin to have trouble breathing while exerting themselves. It is best not to make your body work too hard because it can be due to exercise intolerance and it can cause the adrenalin to run thus causing potassium shifting, and the cycle can begin

Possible Complications

anew; weakening the muscles and organs, which can cause tachycardia and arrhythmia including the long QT interval heartbeat, which can lead cardiac arrest. Or, it may be that one's breathing organs and cardiac muscles are weakening and oxygen therapy may be indicated to ease the excess work of the heart and other organs.

Diagnosing

If an individual with Period Paralysis begins to have breathing problems it would be best to have it checked out with you Primary Care Physician (PCP). The PCP can refer you to a pulmonologist or have your oxygen levels tested using an oximeter with a recorder overnight or for twenty-four hours.

Kidney Issues

Kidney function can be affected in individuals with Periodic Paralysis. We know that when potassium shifts, calcium carbonate from the bone is released. This increase of calcium carbonate, can lead to the formation of kidney stones. We also know if one has chronic metabolic acidosis, as a result of Periodic Paralysis, his or her kidneys can be affected because metabolic acidosis also causes an increase or shifting of potassium into the body fluids causing an increase of calcium carbonate. The use of the commonly used diuretic for patients with Periodic Paralysis, acetazolamide, also known as diamox, can cause kidney stones.

Osteoporosis

When potassium shifts in the body, as it does in Periodic Paralysis, calcium carbonate from the bone is released. This causes a loss of the bone crystals in the bones leading to osteoporosis. Chronic metabolic acidosis, as a result of Periodic Paralysis, also causes the potassium to shift, thus creating bone loss or osteoporosis.

Research indicates there is a connection between Periodic Paralysis and the osteoporosis. Some individuals with Periodic Paralysis can develop early bone loss due to the potassium shifting out of the bones and other organs as it shifts into the muscles. During the shifting, there is a loss of the bone crystals causing bone-loss or osteoporosis.

Metabolic Acidosis/Lactic Acidosis

Metabolic acidosis and lactic acidosis are complex conditions, which can be difficult to understand, but fairly easy to diagnose based on symptoms and lab results. However, in individuals with Periodic Paralysis, they are often overlooked, missed on the lab reports and testing for them is often not requested as a possibility for obvious symptoms. Because Periodic Paralysis is a mineral metabolic disorder and it affects the breathing muscles, individuals with it appear to be susceptible for developing these conditions. Episodes of paralysis are triggered by metabolic and lactic acidosis.

This section, just as the section on heart issues, will be as simplified as possible but some terms will be included which, will be specifically used for recognition and diagnosis by physicians and patients. (More technical information about metabolic acidosis can be found at the end of this chapter.)

Metabolic Acidosis

As we have previously learned, metabolic acidosis is a pH imbalance (the balance between the acid and alkaline), in which the body accumulates an excess of acid in the body fluids and does not have enough bicarbonate to neutralize the effects of the acid effectively. An individual can develop metabolic acidosis, if the carbon dioxide levels are allowed to rise and remain in the body.

We know that metabolic acidosis affects the heart and breathing. It results in potassium shifting out of the cells and into the bloodstream creating hyperkalemia, too much potassium. The combination of metabolic acidosis and hyperkalemia is a serious condition and can be life threatening leading to shock and death.

Symptoms of Metabolic Acidosis

Some of the more common symptoms of metabolic acidosis are muscle weakness, bone and muscle pain, headache, chest pain, tachycardia, heart palpitations, abdominal pain, rapid breathing, shortness of breath, confusion, drowsiness, a lack of energy and paralysis for persons with Periodic Paralysis. If metabolic acidosis becomes severe it can lead to shock (a lack of an appropriate flow of blood in the body) or death. However, the symptoms of metabolic acidosis are sometimes not very obvious or specific, depending on the cause. It should be noted that in some individual's metabolic acidosis could be mild and ongoing (chronic).

In chronic metabolic acidosis an individual's bones and kidneys are affected. When potassium shifts in the body, calcium carbonate from the bone is released. This causes a loss of the bone crystals leading to osteoporosis. When the kidneys are affected and this can be seen by the formation of kidney stones.

Diagnosing Metabolic Acidosis

There are several methods that can be used to diagnose metabolic acidosis; usually more than one will be utilized. The arterial blood gas test is the most important and decisive one used.

The most widely used methods are listed below:

Arterial blood gas: If the pH balance is low (below 7.75) and bicarbonate levels are low, then metabolic acidosis is present.
Anion gap: subtracting chloride and bicarbonate levels from sodium. If elevated (>16 mmol/l) it can indicate metabolic acidosis and lactic acidosis
Serum electrolyte levels (high potassium)
Urine pH: acidity levels
Glucose/sugar levels
Kidney function
Full blood count
An EKG: This will show heart complications such as arrhythmia

Possible Complications

Treatment and Management for Metabolic Acidosis

The best way to treat and manage metabolic acidosis for individuals with Periodic Paralysis is to avoid the causes. It may develop due to an unbalanced diet, exercise or exertion, medications (it should be noted here that diamox or acetazolamide may cause it.), illness, infections or too much potassium, or it may be chronic. Eliminating the medication, avoiding exercise or exertion, eating a balanced pH diet, lowering the level of potassium or treating the infection or illness, will manage the acidosis. Using bicarbonate or increasing alkaline will neutralize the acids. In severe cases, dialysis may be needed. Mechanical assistance or ventilation for breathing may be necessary.

http://livingwithperiodicparalysis.blogspot.com/2013/12/periodic-paralysis-and-metabolic.html

Lactic Acidosis

Lactic acidosis is a form of metabolic acidosis that occurs when blood pH levels in the blood and lactic acid become unbalanced. This is the result of oxygen levels dropping. It forms if the carbohydrates get broken down and are used for energy from the low oxygen levels. The lactic acid increases in the bloodstream more quickly than it can be expelled. Too much lactic acid in the body creates an increase of pyruvic acid. Too much pyruvic acid in the body creates metabolic acid in the body. It can cause mental confusion and lead to a coma. It affects the function of the liver and can develop into multiple organ failure, which can lead to death.

Lactic acidosis can develop in individuals with metabolic disorders, especially ones that do not supply enough oxygen to tissues in the body. This kind is known as Type A lactic acidosis. Because Periodic Paralysis is a disorder in which hypoventilation (slow and shallow breathing) can occur when the breathing muscles weaken, individuals with it, can and do develop metabolic and lactic acidosis.

Lactic acidosis is an indication that there may be mitochondrial damage in the cells from the continual potassium shifting from Periodic Paralysis. This damage of the mitochondria may lead to issues of the autoimmune system leading to autoimmune dysfunction, disorders and diseases.

Symptoms of Lactic Acidosis

Some of the more common symptoms of lactic acidosis are frequent urination or absence of urine output, anemia, low blood pressure, abdominal pain, an enlarged liver, weight loss, breathing problems, hyperventilation, muscle pain, weakness, tiredness, irregular heartbeat, lightheadedness, dizziness, profuse sweating, loss of appetite, nausea, vomiting, headaches, sensitivity to light, moist skin, clammy and cold skin, chills and dry eyes, nose, mouth and throat. As it progresses the hands and feet turn blue, blood pressure drops, heart rate slows, a person feels disoriented and confused and unconsciousness and paralysis sets in for someone with Periodic Paralysis.

Diagnosing Lactic Acidosis

A lactate test is used to determine the amount of lactic acidosis in the blood. The normal values are between 0.5 and 2.2 mmol/L. Above 2.2 (>2.2 mmol/L) would indicate an individual has lactic acidosis. It is best not to use a tourniquet when testing for lactic acidosis because it can cause the results to be falsely elevated.

Treatment and Management for Lactic Acidosis

The best way to treat lactic acidosis is to treat the underlying cause as in metabolic acidosis. In the case of Periodic Paralysis it is best to avoid the causes. It may develop due to an unbalanced diet, exercise or exertion, medications, illness, infections, too much potassium or it may be chronic. Eliminating the medication, avoiding exercise or exertion, eating a balanced pH diet, lowering the level of potassium or treating the infection or illness will manage the acidosis. In severe cases, dialysis may be needed. Mechanical assistance or ventilation for breathing may be necessary. Lactic acidosis may be difficult to avoid in individuals with Periodic Paralysis due to the chronic low oxygen levels from the weak breathing muscles. Oxygen therapy may be necessary.

Pain

Unfortunately, many doctors have the misconception, based on outdated and archaic information and data, that pain is a not a symptom and does not exist in patients who have Periodic Paralysis. This is a serious issue because these doctors refuse to recognize Periodic Paralysis and refuse to diagnose individuals who desperately need to be diagnosed because they experience pain.

Last year we created and carried out a series of four surveys attempting to gather as much information as possible in order to create a set of criteria that doctors could use to aid in diagnosing patients. Ninety-five percent of the participants indicated that they experience pain regardless of their diagnoses; Andersen-Tawil Syndrome, Hypokalemic Periodic Paralysis, Hyperkalemic Periodic Paralysis, Normokalemic Periodic Paralysis or Paramyotonia Congenita. It was the same whether they were diagnosed genetically, clinically or still seeking a diagnosis.

It was discovered that the pain can be experienced before, at the beginning, during or after episodes or it can be intermittent or chronic (all of the time). The pain was described in many ways such as achy, sharp, constant, tenderness, sudden, cramping, rigidity, contractions, tightening, stiffness, charley horses, growing pains or spasms. It was reported as only involving one limb or body part, partial body, the trunk, several body parts or the entire body.

The pain results from several natural ways depending on the type of Periodic Paralysis or genetic mutation. In some cases it is from the swelling of the muscles when they fill up with fluid as the potassium shifts. Some of the pain is from the rigidity and contracting of the muscles. A third cause can be the shifting of sugar with the potassium. A fourth cause may be from low magnesium. Cold can create rigidity and pain for some. Metabolic acidosis, which can often develop in Periodic Paralysis, causes pain in the bones and chest pain.

Other conditions or diseases can co-exist causing permanent or intermittent pain such as Ehlers-Danlos Syndrome (EDS), arthritis or fibromyalgia. These may be aggravated when an individual with Periodic Paralysis is in an episode or paralysis. Intermittent paralytic episodes can damage organs in the body, including the muscles. For some individuals the pain becomes permanent and may be misdiagnosed as fibromyalgia, or other medical issues like rheumatoid arthritis. Pain may also be caused from other unnatural means. The off-label medications typically prescribed for Periodic Paralysis or other drugs such as statins may create pain.

Treatment and Management for Pain

The best method to avoid the pain during the episodes is to avoid the episodes by avoiding the triggers and maintaining a balance in diet, rest, hydration and other natural methods.

Some people with Periodic Paralysis may be able to take medications to ease the pain but many people cannot handle medications. It is advised that the pain be treated with natural means such as eating certain foods, herbal teas, heating pads, warm baths, ice packs, relaxation techniques and massages. More ideas can be found in Chapter Eleven and on the Internet.

http://livingwithperiodicparalysis.blogspot.com/2014/09/pain-and-periodic-paralysis.html

Rhabdomyolysis

Rhabdomyolysis, or muscle wasting, is a serious condition, which is seen in some forms of Periodic Paralysis. It can be caused from low potassium levels. Those with Hypokalemic Periodic Paralysis, especially mutations found in CACNA1S, seem to be more likely to develop it.

In Rhabdomyolysis, skeletal muscle breaks down very quickly. The particles of the damaged muscle enter the bloodstream and are harmful to the kidneys and may cause kidney failure. The symptoms from this can be quite severe including vomiting, pain in the muscles, arrhythmia, tachycardia, confusion and even coma. The more severe the muscle damage, the more serious the symptoms become. Tea-colored urine may develop.

One should seek medical attention immediately.

http://livingwithperiodicparalysis.blogspot.com/2014/02/rhabdomyolysis.html

Drugs and Medications

Paradoxical Reaction and Idiosyncratic Reaction to Drugs

The two most common issues with drugs or pharmaceuticals for individuals with Periodic Paralysis (and others) are a paradoxical reaction and an idiosyncratic reaction. These are both serious effects. If one has a paradoxical reaction to a medication it means that the opposite of what is supposed to happen will occur. For instance, if someone takes a sleeping pill and then stays awake all night, it is known as a paradoxical effect. This can be just an inconvenience or very serious depending on the medical issue and the reaction. If someone who is already experiencing high blood pressure, is prescribed a drug to lower blood pressure, but it increases the blood pressure, this can cause a stroke, other serious effects or even death.

If an individual develops tremors, metabolic acidosis and paralysis from taking an antibiotic; these would be considered as idiosyncratic effects; reactions or side effects, which would be totally unpredicted, unexpected and never seen before. These effects would not be listed as possible rare side effects. This is a serious problem because these idiosyncratic effects, also known as "type B reaction" can be harmful by causing damage or even death. The amount ingested has no bearing on it. The reactions may occur from the smallest amount possible after one dose and the reactions may occur right away or after a little passage of time, even after a few weeks or chronically after a period of time.

It is believed that the type B reaction is an immune-mediated toxicity. This means an idiosyncratic reaction is an immune system response, which causes the drug to be toxic or poisonous to the individual who ingested it, inhaled it or absorbed it through the skin and causes cellular damage. Experience and research indicate that very few treatments exist. One must stop taking the drug, repair the damage if possible and provide life support if needed.

It should be noted that there may be no reaction the first time, but may happen after the second time it is prescribed or at any time, even if taken for many years with no problems. The unexpected reaction may also occur after discontinuing the drug many weeks previously. The reaction or side effect may not be the same each time the drug is introduced.

Research indicates idiosyncratic effects are related to metabolic, mitochondrial and inflammatory dysfunction rather than the immune system and that there might be a genetic link in many cases.

Why is this an issue for individuals with Periodic Paralysis? Periodic Paralysis is a mineral metabolic disorder. Paradoxical reactions and idiosyncratic reactions are related to metabolic dysfunction. Strange, odd and out of the ordinary side effects and drugs creating the opposite effects are common characteristics of individuals with all forms of Periodic Paralysis, especially the form known as Andersen-Tawil Syndrome.

Many individuals with Periodic Paralysis have serious side effects from the drugs they are prescribed. Without knowing this and without a diagnosis, doctors will prescribe drugs to treat symptoms that appear to be neurological or for other issues. The patient will use the pharmaceuticals and develop new symptoms, over time. These symptoms begin to look like something else for which new medications are prescribed, and the cycle continues. Or if there is no diagnosis and a person is suspected of having a conversion disorder, once everything else is ruled out, psychotropic medications may be prescribed. These medications can become out of control and it is not uncommon to be on 5 or 10 or more drugs at one time. They are toxic to the body and are causing damage. Most of them are also triggers for the periods of paralysis, and each paralytic episode causes more damage to the body.

Possible Complications

In conclusion, a paradoxical or idiosyncratic reaction is an immune system response to drugs due to genetic predisposition and metabolic dysfunction in individuals with Periodic Paralysis, a mineral metabolic disorder. This includes the medications specifically prescribed to treat Periodic Paralysis. Precautions must be taken to avoid these effects. Stop the drugs or do not start them at all. There are natural ways to control many of the symptoms of Periodic Paralysis, namely avoiding triggers and other common sense and natural methods.

http://livingwithperiodicparalysis.blogspot.com/2013/12/idiosyncratic-and-paradoxical-reactions.html
http://en.wikipedia.org/wiki/Idiosyncratic_drug_reaction
http://en.wikipedia.org/wiki/Toxicology

Acetazolamide-Diamox

One of the major drugs used for treating Periodic Paralysis is acetazolamide, also sold under the name of diamox. It is an off-label drug, which means this drug is made and used to treat conditions other than Periodic Paralysis. The fact is there are NO drugs recommended or approved by the Food and Drug Administration (FDA) to treat Periodic Paralysis. It is a carbonic anhydrase inhibitor, which is a diuretic. It removes water through the kidneys. Interestingly, it is used to treat mild metabolic acidosis (discussed above), however, it actually leads to more metabolic acidosis by speeding up the process. Many individuals taking this drug to treat their symptoms of Periodic Paralysis are unknowingly making themselves worse and causing more damage to their bodies. It also lowers potassium so it is questionable for use with Hypokalemic Periodic Paralysis. It is also linked to permanent muscle weakness. Many people are also unaware that it is a sulfa-based drug and should not be taken if an allergy exists to sulfa drugs.

If one already has Periodic Paralysis and has chronic metabolic acidosis he or she can develop kidney stones and osteoporosis over time. If one already has Periodic Paralysis and has chronic metabolic acidosis and takes diamox, he or she can become more acidic and can acquire full blown metabolic acidosis which causes more damage and kidney stones and accelerates osteoporosis, more illness, more paralysis from the stress on the body and lowering of potassium and may even cause death.

There are also warnings about children using acetazolamide. The safety and effectiveness have not even been tested for those under twelve. There are three major side effects seen in children; 'fits,' growth retardation and weakening of the bones.

Research indicates that only 50% of those with Hypokalemic Periodic Paralysis, especially with the SCN4A genetic mutation, do not respond to acetazolamide and it may actually cause paralysis or worse symptoms. So, if someone is diagnosed with Hypokalemic Periodic Paralysis, they must be very careful, it should be used with extreme caution. It should not automatically be given to people who are clinically diagnosed with Hypokalemic Periodic Paralysis or if it is, it should be monitored closely.

About half of the individuals with Periodic Paralysis do not have a genetic diagnosis and do not know what sequence or genetic mutation they actually have. Further study and research are recommended before taking it so you will know what to expect or what to look for, in order to be safe.

Some do well on this medication. If it is working and there are no side effects, then there are no problems. If, however, this drug may be causing side effects or if one is attempting to decide whether to take it or not, hopefully this information can help in making an informed decision.

http://livingwithperiodicparalysis.blogspot.com/2014/02/some-forms-of-pp-worsened-by-diamox.html
http://www.periodicparalysisnetwork.com/pdf/Metabolic%20Acidosis%20Article.pdf
http://livingwithperiodicparalysis.blogspot.com/2013/12/periodic-paralysis-and-metabolic.html
http://livingwithperiodicparalysis.blogspot.com/2014/06/beware-of-off-label-drugs.html

Intravenous Therapy (IV's)

One of the greatest fears individuals with Periodic Paralysis have is ending up in the ER at the mercy of doctors who do not understand the condition while they are in full body paralysis. The first the medical professionals want to do is attach an IV, short for intravenous therapy. This is frightening because they can be a serious trigger for most forms of Periodic Paralysis. IV's of glucose or dextrose (sugar and water), or saline or sodium (salt and water) can create paralysis; make an episode worse and in some cases cause death.

If an IV is needed in an emergency situation, for severely low potassium, mannitol may be used in diluted strengths and only small amounts every twenty to sixty minutes. Hyperkalemia may develop otherwise. Close monitoring of the heart and potassium levels are necessary. It must be used with great care because it is also dehydrating.

Individuals with Hyperkalemic Periodic Paralysis may benefit from the use of a glucose IV.

Individuals with Periodic Paralysis have used Hartmann's IV Solution with some success. It may be a good option, especially if acidosis is present. It contains a mixture of electrolytes.

Many individuals with Periodic Paralysis are made to endure pain, more paralysis, harm and sometimes-even death due to doctors not listening to the patients or their family members about this serious issue.

http://livingwithperiodicparalysis.blogspot.com/2013/12/why-people-with-some-forms-of-periodic.html

Anesthesia

As previously discussed, Periodic Paralysis is a mineral metabolic disorder, also known as an ion channelopathy, which is a dysfunction of the ion channels. The ion channels transport the electrolytes, such as sodium and potassium through the cells. This transport is faulty in individuals with ion channel dysfunction and extreme care must be used when anesthesia is going to be utilized. This is due to the possibility of developing serious symptoms such as breathing issues or failure, arrhythmia, blood pressure issues, choking, muscle weakness or paralysis, longer recovery after surgery, malignant hyperthermia or death. Managing the use of anesthesia in individuals with Periodic Paralysis is mostly aimed at preventing attacks of paralysis or the other symptoms during

Possible Complications

or after surgery. The manner in which the situation is handled for the individual depends on which form of Periodic Paralysis is involved.

Malignant Hyperthermia (MH): As mentioned previously, individuals with Periodic Paralysis are at risk for developing malignant hyperthermia during or after surgery. All forms of Periodic Paralysis are the result of mutations on Chromosome 17. Malignant hyperthermia is also the result of a mutation on Chromosome 17, thus creating the potential for those with Periodic Paralysis, including, Normokalemic Periodic Paralysis, to develop the serious and life-threatening symptoms involved with the use of anesthesia.

Hypokalemic Periodic Paralysis and Anesthesia: For individuals with Hypokalemic Periodic Paralysis, anesthesia is a known trigger for paralytic episodes. According to research, in order to successfully manage the patient there is need for an evaluation before surgery, avoidance of known triggers, careful monitoring during the surgery and immediate and proper treatment if an issue arises.

Hyperkalemic Periodic Paralysis and Anesthesia: Nothing was written about the use of anesthesia and Hyperkalemic Periodic Paralysis before 2002. Early research concluded that anesthesia might be used without complications if the potassium levels were with-in normal levels prior to surgery, if the carbohydrate levels were up, if anesthetic drugs, which released potassium, were not used and if normal body temperature levels were maintained.

Andersen-Tawil Syndrome and Anesthesia: Some research indicated that malignant hyperthermia is not usually an issue for individuals with Andersen-Tawil Syndrome. However, it is an issue because individuals with ATS have shifting of potassium into both high and low ranges causing symptoms and paralysis. The other issue with anesthesia use and ATS is a need for special precautions due to the serious issue of the long QT interval heartbeat, a diagnostic marker for the condition and torsades de pointes another extremely serious arrhythmia. There are many medications that must be avoided, which are used routinely in preparation for surgery and during surgery including the glucose and sodium IVs, as well as most forms of anesthesia.

Lidocaine: Topical, regional and local anesthesia may cause potassium to drop in individuals with Hypokalemic Periodic Paralysis, Normokalemic Periodic Paralysis or Andersen-Tawil Syndrome if it contains epinephrine. The most often discussed and utilized local anesthesia is lidocaine. For some individuals it may work well if the epinephrine is removed. For others it may cause hypokalemia or arrhythmia regardless of the epinephrine being removed. For others still, it may not work at all or the usual amount may be needed during a procedure. Lidocaine and other local types of anesthesia need to be used with extreme caution.

Anyone with Periodic Paralysis needs to be extremely cautious when planning any surgical procedures, which may use anesthesia.

More Information: More specific information is written about Periodic Paralysis and the use of anesthesia, but due to copyright laws it is not included in this book. The article was written and created with a compilation of information, excerpts, references and links related to the problems and issues of the use of anesthesia with individuals with the various forms of Periodic Paralysis. There is quite a bit of technical information, which can be shared with your doctor, anesthesiologist or dentist (though most of them should know this information). Please visit this blog and copy it and place it in your personal medical journal for future reference.

http://livingwithperiodicparalysis.blogspot.com/2014/02/periodic-paralysis-and-anesthesia.html

No Tourniquet

Another complication that needs to be included here is related to the drawing of blood for measuring potassium levels in the blood. It is recommended that a tourniquet should not be used. When blood is drawn using a tourniquet it can result in potassium levels, which are higher than they really are. It is important to understand that improper use of a tourniquet and the clenching of the fist can result in false lab results for potassium levels. The pressure (too tight) and time (too long) of the tourniquet can raise the level of potassium as much as 10% to 20%. This difference can be important when making a decision about treatment or trying to get diagnosed.

More specific and technical information and links are found in the following article. It would be wise to copy the article and like the anesthesia article, add it to your personal medical journal for future reference and to share when drawing blood for potassium levels are necessary.

http://livingwithperiodicparalysis.blogspot.com/2014/02/no-tourniquet-please.html

As explained at the beginning of this chapter, many complications are associated with Periodic Paralysis, especially when the condition has been misdiagnosed and mistreated over a period of many years. The next chapter will discuss more complex issues and obstacles related to this condition.

Five
More Complications
UNDERSTAND THE COMPLEXITY

Several other forms of complications, confusion, difficulty and obstacles exist for recognition, diagnosis and treatment related to Periodic Paralysis. These are more complex and multifaceted than those discussed previously. They are serious, seldom discussed and most certainly overlooked.

Co-Existing Conditions

The term 'co-existing conditions' also known as 'co-morbidity' means having more than one medical condition, illness or disease at the same time. Last year we prepared and executed a comprehensive four-part informal survey of the members of our Periodic Paralysis Network Support Group and received a great deal of important and surprising information. We discovered that most of our members had more than just the common symptoms of Periodic Paralysis. Many of them, whether they were diagnosed with a form of Periodic Paralysis or not, had at least one more other diagnosed condition. Most had several, and a few had as many as fifteen other diagnosed diseases, conditions or types of medical dysfunction. The following is the list of conditions reported:

Cyclic vomiting syndrome, high cholesterol, diabetes type 2, peripheral polyneuropathy, arachnoids cysts in the brain, loss of peripheral vision, poly cystic ovarian disease, migraines, osteoporosis (bone crush stage in spine and hips), spina bifida oculta, small brain ischemia, intolerance to most medications, paradoxical effect to most medications, hypoglycemia, intolerance to anesthesia, cataracts, costochondritis, gluten intolerance, fibrocystic disease, esophageal reflux, esophageal hernia, diverticulitis, hearing loss, lactic acidosis, metabolic acidosis, hypoxemia, (low blood oxygen), restless leg syndrome, stress fracture of the foot, neuroma (nerve tumor) in both feet, painful and tight calf muscles, fibroid tumor (uterus), ovarian cysts, chronic bladder infections, extremely dry skin, GERD, weak eye muscles, fasciculations, temporomandibular disorders, reflex sympathetic dystrophy, cervical and uterine cancer, uterine and ovarian cysts, vertigo, high clotting, blood clots, asthma, low set, hyper mobile joints, gastritis, syncope, muscle spasms, depression, obsessive compulsive disorder, memory loss (short term), chronic fatigue, edema, unnamed lumps in breasts, herpes simplex A (lips-cold sores), gastro paresis, myalgia, myositis, osteoarthritis, myoclonic jerks, dysphagia (trouble swallowing), lumbar spinal stenosis, many cysts, fatty tumors, hyperthyroid, clotting disorder, memory deficit, compressed pituitary, kidney cyst, allergies, goiter, hardening of the arteries in legs, trouble climbing stairs, low platelet count, mastectomy and hysterectomy, straight spine, vertigo, tinnitus, atrial septal defect, complete heart block, scoliosis, pitting edema, thyroid hormone resistance disease, seizures, cluster headaches, severe sleep apnea, rectocele, pulmonary hypertension, candida, acute pancreatitis, chronic pancreatitis, poorly distended bladder, Barrett's esophagus, migraines, heart attack, gall bladder issues, carpal tunnel, exercise intolerance, kidney stones, degenerative disk disease, Ehlers-Danlos Syndrome, fibromyalgia, interstitial cystitis, Sjogrens Syndrome, LUPUS, Charcot-Marie Tooth.

The Periodic Paralysis Guide And Workbook

We know that some of these conditions are related to other mutations on chromosome 17, the same chromosome responsible for several forms of Periodic Paralysis. Individuals with genetic mutations on Chromosome 17 may also be susceptible to other conditions on the same chromosome. (It should also be noted that forms of Periodic Paralysis found on other chromosomes might also have this susceptibility.) These are often called 'sister' conditions or diseases. Apparently, if one has a mutation on a particular chromosome, they may also have other conditions, which can be found on that chromosome. For instance, an individual with Hypokalemic Periodic Paralysis found at SCN4A on chromosome 17 may also have one or more of over eighty conditions including the following: Malignant Hyperthermia, Ehler-Danlos Syndrome (EDS), Familial Atrial Fibrillation, Glycogen Storage Disease, Lamb-Girdle Muscular Dystrophy, Paramyotonia Congenita, Potassium-Aggravated Myotonia and even other forms of Periodic Paralysis.

We also now know, through research, that some of the other symptoms, diseases and conditions are likely to be related to the Periodic Paralysis. Many of the above conditions are also ion channelopathies, forms of metabolic disorder. They include: fibromyalgia, malignant hyperthermia, chronic fatigue, long QT syndrome, seizures, congenital hypoglycemia, inherited cardiac arrhythmia, migraines, involuntary movement, epilepsy, some autoimmune diseases and hypertension.

We learned that our members, besides having some or all of the complications listed and possible "sister" conditions, they also have any combination of allergies, autoimmune and inflammatory diseases, conditions and dysfunction (all autoimmune) and even some mitochondrial dysfunction. Also revealed was what appeared to be a correlation between the length of time an individual had gone without a diagnosis and proper treatment, the number of complications and co-existing conditions they had. Age also played a factor. For many, the older the person, the more other complications and conditions existed.

More results from the survey indicated that the individuals who had the most co-morbidity had the symptoms of Periodic Paralysis the longest without proper treatment and without a diagnosis. They had been treated with improper or unnecessary drugs. They had more co-existing diseases and conditions and more overall disability and permanent muscle weakness. The other group of individuals with more co-existing conditions was the children of parents who also had Periodic Paralysis. In many, each generation seemed to experience more severe symptoms than the previous generation.

Through further research it was discovered that Periodic Paralysis, a mineral metabolic disorder, could cause damage to the mitochondria in the cells. (This may be due to the atypical shifting of potassium.) The damage to the DNA of the mitochondria, in turn contributes to the development of autoimmune disorders. It is our hope that more research will be done in this area, to better be able to recognize and diagnose Periodic Paralysis even though it may co-existing with other conditions and diseases.

Unfortunately, the Periodic Paralysis 'specialists' and the 'purists' have not recognized these connections and therefore refuse to diagnose individuals who have diseases or conditions co-existing with the symptoms of Periodic Paralysis. It appears the more conditions that develop; the more difficult it is to recognize the Periodic Paralysis.

More Complications

Periodic Paralysis Plus 10 Syndrome (PP+10S)

In our first book we discussed the possibility of a new form of Periodic Paralysis that we named Periodic Paralysis Plus 10 Syndrome (PP+10S). Most of our members at that time had similar symptoms that were outside of the normal symptoms described in all of the literature and some many had characteristics similar to those seen in Andersen-Tawil Syndrome.

First, as described in the book, although none of the individuals at that time had a known genetic mutation that had been discovered yet, though many of them were diagnosed clinically, they all had symptoms of periods of paralysis, total and/or partial, which involved the shifting of potassium, either, up, down or in normal ranges.

Next, most had symptoms of blood pressure changes during them, which can be up or down or fluctuating. They also have heart arrhythmia (some long QT) and tachycardia or bradycardia or both during the attacks. Most had problems breathing and some with choking. (These fit the ATS description. It certainly appeared ATS-like.)

Third, the majority of the members had at least ten other identified and diagnosed conditions, which were the same. The conditions, which appeared over and over again in each one of them, were:

- Fibromyalgia/Chronic Fatigue
- Osteoarthritis
- Degenerative disk disease
- Heart problems, tachycardia, bradycardia, arrhythmia,
- Long QT
- Pain disorders
- Blood pressure problems, (high or low)
- Sleep disorders, (insomnia, sleep apnea)
- Constipation (hemorrhoids)
- Exercise intolerance
- Female organ dysfunctions

Fourth, nearly every member had one or more of the over one hundred conditions and diseases, listed in the previous section, co-existing with their Periodic Paralysis symptoms.

After completing the four-part survey, studying the results and researching these issues, (once the first book was written), we found some answers, which may explain the facts we uncovered and which may help with the development of a new method to diagnose Periodic Paralysis. It appears there is a Periodic Paralysis Plus Ten Syndrome but not in the way that we first expected it to be. It actually encompasses every form of Periodic Paralysis.

The interesting thing we first discovered was that there is not much difference between symptoms of the three main types whether diagnosed genetically, clinically or those still waiting for a diagnosis!

The survey results indicated that of the sixty-one members, who participated, 18% had a genetic diagnosis, 51% had a clinical diagnosis and 31% had no diagnosis. The results were the same, however. All but one individual (which was controlled by drugs) had symptoms of intermittent paralysis, total and/or partial, which involved the shifting of potassium, either, up, down or in normal ranges.

The symptoms involved with blood pressure changes, which can be up or down or fluctuating; heart arrhythmia and tachycardia or bradycardia or both during the attacks; breathing issues and some choking all happened during paralytic episodes for all forms of Periodic Paralysis. They were not exclusive to ATS. However, the levels of blood pressure, the types of arrhythmia and other symptoms were different depending on the form of Periodic Paralysis.

Of the original ten co-existing conditions, the heart and blood pressure issues proved to be normal parts of the paralytic episodes as was constipation. Pain affected 95% of the members and 90% experienced exercise intolerance an example of progression of the condition, both of which were normal complications for Periodic Paralysis. The remaining five fell under the category 'sister' diseases, other ion channelopathies, and any combination of allergies, autoimmune and auto inflammatory diseases, conditions and dysfunction (all autoimmune) and mitochondrial dysfunction.

Typically, the longer one had the symptoms of Periodic Paralysis (the older they are) or from when the symptoms started, and those who were left untreated the longest, the more likely they were to have the complications which can be seen as 'natural progression' or 'levels' of the condition, mitochondrial, auto inflammatory and autoimmune issues.

Also worth noting was that 92% of the members reported at least one ATS characteristic (discussed later in this chapter) despite the form of Periodic Paralysis they were diagnosed with either genetically, clinically or those with no diagnosis. This led to the speculation that many of the ATS characteristics are either seen in normal individuals on a regular basis, or the characteristics, which are supposed to be unique to ATS, are also seen in other forms of Periodic Paralysis, but in a more subtle manner or have just been overlooked in the original research of patients with other forms of Periodic Paralysis.

Based on all of the above information, we are purposing a new, sensible, practical and more reliable way to diagnose Periodic Paralysis; a checklist that includes the type of Periodic Paralysis based on the symptoms, degree of progression or 'level', and the 'stage' to which it has developed. This method will take away the issue of withholding a diagnosis based on coexisting conditions such as autoimmune disorders, or mitochondrial dysfunction, because they are actually a part of the process of Periodic Paralysis over a lifetime. They are an indication of the stage of the Periodic Paralysis. It is simply the level and stage, which has developed in the individual due to non-treatment, improper treatment or treatment that does not work and non-diagnosis. The stages we developed are as follows:

More Complications

Stage of Periodic Paralysis:

Stage One=periods of muscle weakness, or partial or full-body paralysis

Stage Two=periods of muscle weakness, or partial or full-body paralysis and PP+ 1-10 (or more)

Stage Three= periods of muscle weakness, or partial or full-body paralysis and PP+ 1-10 (or more) and Autoimmune Dysfunction

Stage Four=periods of muscle weakness, or partial or full-body paralysis and PP+ 1-10 (or more) and Mitochondrial Dysfunction

Stage Five=periods of muscle weakness, or partial or full-body paralysis and PP+ 1-10 (or more) and Mitochondrial Dysfunction and Autoimmune Dysfunction

To explain this I will use my own symptoms to illustrate the process. I have periods of paralysis from low, high and normal potassium levels with long QT interval heartbeats. I have Andersen-Tawil Syndrome (ATS) and Paramyotonia Congenita (PMC). I have 18 coexisting conditions, which include mitochondrial issues (lactic acidosis) and autoimmune disorders (fibromyalgia, celiac disease, allergies, diabetes, restless leg syndrome and more) (PP+18). I have progressive conditions and complications, including progressive muscle weakness, exercise intolerance and permanent heart issues. My degree of progression or level is (DP/L4). My stage is 5.

My diagnosis will be written out as: **ATS&PMC, PP+18, DP or Level 4, Stage 5**

This formula is very clear to understand. It is sensible, practical and a more reliable way to diagnose Periodic Paralysis. Looking at it indicates I have ATS, I have 18 coexisting conditions, the degree of progression is at level 4 out of 4 and the stage I am now at is 5 out of 5. It is easy to see that I am old, very, very ill and have progressed to a very advanced stage due to a lifetime of misdiagnoses, mis treatments, wrong and unnecessary drugs and inability to use medications, which could improve some of the conditions. Another diagnosis formula might look like this: **HypoPP, PP+2, DP or level 0, Stage 1**.

It is easy to see that this individual is either young or has been using medication that helps, or is following the plans to better manage his or her symptoms.

The diagnosis and proper treatment of all the forms of Periodic Paralysis in a timely manner is absolutely imperative in order to avoid the possible complications including mitochondrial damage and autoimmune dysfunction and to slow or stop the progression of the disease, which can be permanent.

More about diagnosing Periodic Paralysis is found in Chapter Thirteen as well a chart for using this new method.

The Periodic Paralysis Guide And Workbook

ATS-like Characteristics of Periodic Paralysis

Andersen-Tawil Syndrome (ATS) is the most rare form of Periodic Paralysis. It accounts for approximately 10% of all periodic paralysis cases. It is characterized by three particular components: periods of paralysis from high, low or normal potassium levels, distinctive craniofacial and skeletal characteristics and long QT interval heartbeat with a predisposition toward life-threatening ventricular arrhythmia. However, affected individuals may express only one or two of the three components and they may be very subtle. Other characteristics and abnormalities are also associated with Andersen-Tawil Syndrome.

These physical abnormalities and characteristics, which are associated with Andersen-Tawil Syndrome, are found on page twenty-four.

Although these characteristics are associated specifically with Andersen-Tawil Syndrome, the survey results for this category were very surprising. The majority, 92% of the members, reported at least one ATS characteristic despite the fact that only two members were diagnosed genetically and two members were diagnosed clinically. This also included members who were genetically diagnosed with the other forms of Periodic Paralysis. The majority of these characteristics were related to the fingers, toes and facial features. Many of the members shared photos of these anomalies. The photos were stunning. Compared to the photos in the medical journals, our members had much more pronounced curved little fingers and webbed 2-3 toes and craniofacial features.

These findings could not be dismissed as a coincidence. There is a strong possibility that many of the ATS characteristics are quite possibly also seen in the other forms of Periodic Paralysis. Is it possible that these features or traits may have been overlooked in the previous research of patients with other types of Periodic Paralysis?

For this reason, we are including these traits or characteristics as possible more in-depth complications and they may be added to the list of symptoms and characteristics for clinically diagnosing all forms of Periodic Paralysis. This may be essential due to the complications some of these features, like scoliosis, dental anomalies, joint laxity, small jaws or issues with executive functioning may pose.

http://livingwithperiodicparalysis.blogspot.com/2013/12/what-is-andersen-tawil-syndrome.html

The Normokalemic Dilemma

The commonly accepted range for normal potassium in human beings is 3.5 to 5.0 mEq/l (milliequivalents per liter), but these numbers may vary somewhat among labs. Our bodies work to naturally maintain a fine balance, which is within that normal range. Ninety-eight percent of potassium in the body is located within the cells and the other two percent of potassium is outside of the cells in the blood. Blood testing in a lab is used to measure the potassium in the body. There are also a few different types of potassium readers available for purchase and use in the home.

More Complications

For individuals with Periodic Paralysis, the 'normal' ranges of potassium may vary significantly from person to person. Results from the survey revealed some feel well and are at their best at about 5.0 while others may do best at 3.8 or 4.3. The potassium, for these individuals, shifts in several ways depending on the type of Periodic Paralysis, causing many symptoms as discussed elsewhere in this book. It may shift higher or lower. These shifts may be very slight yet cause paralysis as well as other serious symptoms including but not limited to heart, breathing and blood pressure issues. The shifting may also happen very quickly and be undetectable. This shifting is then within the 'normal' ranges of potassium, thus the name 'Normokalemic' Periodic Paralysis, although some research indicates it is not necessarily a distinct or different form of Periodic Paralysis, but rather Hyperkalemic Periodic Paralysis. However, it appears that 58% of those surveyed with all forms of PP actually have episodes of potassium shifting within normal ranges according to a recent survey of individuals diagnosed genetically and clinically.

Because most of the emphasis, literature and studies written about Periodic Paralysis are about Hypokalemic Periodic Paralysis (low potassium) and Hyperkalemic Periodic Paralysis (high potassium), the majority of medical professionals do not understand or recognize Normokalemic Periodic Paralysis or the knowledge that the potassium does not have to shift outside of normal ranges or that it may shift too quickly to be detected to create the paralysis or other symptoms which may be serious or life-threatening. It may also shift high or low and return to normal ranges before an individual can be tested in a lab or be seen in the ER.

This makes it difficult when an individual is seeking a diagnosis. Neurologists suspect neurological issues and prescribe very harmful medications, which may cause new symptoms or physical therapy, which can be painful and cause episodes of paralysis. Unfortunately, this may then lead to misdiagnoses of pseudo-seizures, conversion disorder, malingering, attention seeking, and/or hypochondria. More inappropriate and harmful medications and treatments are prescribed to treat these issues. The mis-labels follow the patient from doctor to doctor and the individual is never taken seriously.

These same issues are rampant in an ER situation. Potassium in normal ranges, with paralysis and other issues and uninformed medical professionals, can add up to all of the above and the administration of IV's which are filled with sodium or glucose with a psychotropic drug to treat pseudo seizures. This can lead to more serious symptoms, permanent damage and even death for an individual with Periodic Paralysis.

Another problem resulting from potassium shifting within normal ranges for someone who has a diagnosis of Periodic Paralysis, especially Hypokalemic Periodic Paralysis (low potassium), is the issues of automatically taking a dose of potassium when symptoms begin or being given an IV with potassium in the ER when the potassium never left normal range. This may then cause a shift into high potassium levels and create new or worse symptoms.

For those who have symptoms and paralysis while potassium levels remain within normal ranges, the best way to know how to treat it is to take note of the symptoms and record them. If one is able to record the levels of potassium at home, keeping a running tally when symptoms begin will eventually show either a trend toward high or low potassium or a shifting both ways as is common in ATS. Depending on whether one gets better or worse when taking potassium, may also be a clue of either high or low potassium. Discovering and avoiding the triggers that set it off is recommended.

http://livingwithperiodicparalysis.blogspot.com/2014/02/what-is-normokalemic-periodic-paralysis.html

Wikipedia. (October 2014). Periodic Paralysis. Retrieved from: http://en.wikipedia.org/wiki/Periodic_paralysis

Conversion Disorder vs. Periodic Paralysis

The term 'conversion disorder' (a mental illness) comes up often in conversation among individuals who have Periodic Paralysis. Many have been victims of this mislabel. Due to the potential harm and detriment that this unfortunate diagnosis may bring to the individual with Periodic Paralysis, we have chosen to include it in this chapter about complications. With each wrong diagnosis, serious and life-threatening complications may arise. Wrong medications due to this unforgivable and unfortunate mistake may be prescribed. Due to a lack of proper treatment, patients get sicker, more damage is done to the organs, permanent muscle weakness sets in and death may occur. This is called iatrogenesis, illness caused directly from a doctor's treatment or lack of appropriate treatment.

Statistics indicate it takes approximately twenty years for someone to get a diagnosis for Periodic Paralysis. This is inexcusable and is due to several factors. First, everything else must be ruled out and secondly, because it looks "fake" to doctors. One of the physicians, who originally diagnosed me, told me that of the few patients he has had with Periodic Paralysis, they were all diagnosed with 'conversion disorder' before they got their diagnosis. I myself received this diagnosis, as did many of the 300 members of the Periodic Paralysis Network Support, Education and Advocacy Group.

This did not happen a hundred or even fifty years ago, but happens daily. A few months ago, one young woman went into full body paralysis lasting many frightening hours. She came out of it to discover she was in such a weakened state that she could not walk or even do something as simple as get dressed without becoming totally fatigued and she was in total body pain. Doctors evaluated her and sent her to a psychiatrist. She was diagnosed with conversion disorder and prescribed a well-known drug used to treat depressive disorders and a well-known pain reliever. She spent the next few months unable to walk and in excruciating pain and in and out of paralytic attacks each lasting many hours. She was unable to work or take care of her young children.

Upon learning of Periodic Paralysis (PP), after much research, her husband discovered the effects of the drugs on someone with PP. He found out that both medications had elements that can actually trigger the paralytic episodes. Immediately she began to taper off of them. Within weeks, pain began to ease; she was able to stand and walk a few steps with help and became somewhat functional again. After a few more weeks she was walking with the aid of two canes and able to do simple tasks. She did not have any episodes of paralysis for two months. Though she does not have a diagnosis and probably will not get one for some time to come, her psychiatrist now regrets his diagnosis and prescribing the drugs. He has been referred for more tests to possibly diagnose Periodic Paralysis.

Another patient, an older man, has suffered with paralytic episodes for years. Gradual muscle weakness ensued until this person had to give up a teaching career. Testing ruled everything else out and a muscle biopsy revealed damage to muscle fibers consistent with PP. Despite these findings, after being forced to see a psychiatrist, the man was diagnosed with conversion disorder while in the hospital because of almost constant paralytic episodes.

This is just the tip of the iceberg for individuals with Periodic Paralysis. They have unexplained bouts with partial to total body paralysis, which include frightening heart arrhythmia; choking; fluctuating blood pressure and heart rate. While in this state they are unable to communicate, they are given IV's with medications/drugs/compounds, which make it worse. They are able to hear everything going on as the doctors insist they are faking it, insisting they are having pseudo seizures, pinching them or sticking them with needles to make them respond, demeaning and insulting them and their family members. Conversion disorder is written in the charts and comments like, "refused to lift leg when asked" was written rather than the truth, which was "cannot lift his leg when asked." Some people actually die during these horrific ER or hospital stays and the death certificate may contain any number of false causes.

To learn more about conversion disorder and iatrogenic treatment go to:

http://livingwithperiodicparalysis.blogspot.com/2013/12/conversion-disorder-vs-periodic.html

http://livingwithperiodicparalysis.blogspot.com/2013/11/periodic-paralysis-and-iatrogenic.html

Conclusion

Most material written about Periodic Paralysis is very simple, basic and limited. That is, there are several forms and the symptoms; usually episodes of paralysis or muscles weakness, occur due to the improper shifting of potassium. Taking potassium can stop episodes or prevent them and most people live a normal life span without complications. This chapter demonstrates that Periodic Paralysis is much more complex and multifaceted than previously written about in most articles and publications and shared by most researchers and doctors. Many of these complications, issues, symptoms and characteristics are very serious, overlooked and rarely discussed. They need to be recognized and used as part of the diagnostic and treatment process.

More detailed information about every aspect of Periodic Paralysis can be found throughout this guide, in our book *living with Periodic Paralysis: The Mystery Unraveled*, on our website and on our blog.

Section II
The Plan

Six
The Plan
THE OUTLINE

Chapter Six outlines the plan or method we call 'walking the tightrope' and the remainder of this book will go into great detail and expand on each component including how to discover your triggers, how to relieve your symptoms, how to get a diagnosis, how to find a doctor, how to monitor the symptoms and much more.

While seeking relief of my own symptoms, these methods were created after much trial and error for the treatment and management for a variant of Andersen-Tawil Syndrome and Paramyotonia Congenita. Others with varying forms of Periodic Paralysis, using these methods, have also found success by individualizing the plan for their specific form of Periodic Paralysis. We call it 'walking a tightrope' because it is a fine balance we must walk to manage our symptoms and avoid paralysis. Every step or component must be strictly followed and adhered to or it will not work. Each step depends on the one before it and the one following it. One misstep can set everything into motion once again. An individual will become out of balance and paralytic episodes and other symptoms will repeatedly occur. In other words, one may fall off of the 'tightrope.'

This method or plan can be modified and individualized for each person with Periodic Paralysis. No doctors assisted in this endeavor and much of the information was gleaned from the Internet and in discussion with people who experience Periodic Paralysis, Paramyotonia Congenita and Andersen-Tawil Syndrome. Each component will be discussed and elaborated on in the following chapters.

Each plan is written in steps including goals and objectives; a list of distinct and separate steps in a task analysis format and the methods to achieve success are explained and described and tools such as charts are included.

The Outline
How To Treat, Control and Manage Periodic Paralysis?

- ❖ Educate Yourself
    - ➢ Join a Periodic Paralysis Community
    - ➢ Search the Internet
    - ➢ Read books

- ❖ Monitor Your Vitals
    - ➢ Obtain medical equipment
        - Cardy meter
        - Oximeter
        - Stethoscope
        - Wrist blood pressure device
        - Ear thermometer
        - PH monitor
        - Blood sugar monitor

- ❖ Know And Understand Your Symptoms
  - ➢ Identify paralysis episodes
  - ➢ Identify other symptoms
  - ➢ Chart symptoms

- ❖ Identify And Eliminate All Known Triggers
  - ➢ Record symptoms and possible causes
  - ➢ Monitor symptoms
  - ➢ Keep a journal

- ❖ Relieve Your Symptoms
  - ➢ Avoid all known triggers
    - Medications
    - Stress
  - ➢ Eat a pH balanced diet
  - ➢ Avoid processed foods
  - ➢ Use organic foods
  - ➢ Drink distilled water
  - ➢ Use organic natural supplements
  - ➢ Stay well rested
  - ➢ Stay well hydrated
  - ➢ Avoid physical exercise and exertion
  - ➢ Avoid heat and cold
  - ➢ Treating paralysis
    - Take potassium or not
    - Take glucose or carbohydrates or not
    - Use oxygen during paralysis
    - Do nothing
  - ➢ Use meditation and mental image

- ❖ Finding a Doctor
  - ➢ Ask present doctors for names of doctors
  - ➢ Ask present doctors for referrals to doctors who may know about PP
  - ➢ Call insurance company
  - ➢ Call doctors' offices
  - ➢ Research on the Internet
  - ➢ Contact the nearest MDA office to get a referral
  - ➢ Think "outside the box"
  - ➢ Be creative

- ❖ Getting a Diagnosis
  - ➢ Process of elimination
    - Gather the facts
      - Lab work
      - Periods of paralysis, documented
      - EKG's.
      - Oximeter recordings

The Plan

- Testing
- Previous medical records
- Chart the triggers
- Document potassium use
- Gather and chart family information

❖ Getting Proper Medical Treatment
  ➢ Assemble a team of doctors (knowledgeable about PP or willing to learn)
    - PCP
    - Neurologist
    - Electrocardiologist
    - Nephrologist
    - Endocrinologist
    - Counselor or therapist
    - Others as needed for symptoms
    - MDA doctors
  ➢ Direct the team
    - Primary Care Doctor
    - Paramedics
    - Emergency Rooms and Hospital Staff

Notes _____
_____
_____
_____
_____
_____
_____
_____
_____
_____
_____
_____
_____
_____
_____
_____
_____
_____
_____
_____
_____
_____
_____
_____

Seven
Educate Yourself
DISCUSSION GROUPS, WEBSITES, INTERNET AND BOOKS

- ❖ **Educate Yourself**
  - ➢ **Join a Periodic Paralysis Community**
  - ➢ **Search the Internet**
  - ➢ **Read books**

If a person has been diagnosed with a form of Periodic Paralysis, whether it is by the discovery of a DNA mutation, by clinical means (which is based on symptoms) or self-diagnosis, they should learn everything they are able to about every aspect of the disorder. It is also necessary that they educate their family members and friends. Knowing about and understanding the syndrome will ease fears and assist with proper diagnosis, management and treatment. Also the knowledge that other people will aid the patient during paralytic episodes can ease the fears.

Joining a Periodic Paralysis discussion or support group or board on the Internet is one of the best methods to discover information about Periodic Paralysis. Being part of a Periodic Paralysis community is vital. You will know that you not alone. You will receive encouragement, support, empathy and sympathy when needed. You will gain information and knowledge from other people who live with the same condition and symptoms on a daily basis. People ask questions and share information. There are several types of groups. Some groups are called listservs, which allow you to post questions and get answers using email. Some groups are Facebook pages. Some groups are specific to the type of Periodic Paralysis, like Familial Hypokalemic Periodic Paralysis. Some are for individuals with all forms of Periodic Paralysis and some are specific to and restricted to only people who have a known genetic mutation. Some have doctors who will answer questions, though they do not always respond or do not respond in a timely manner.

The Periodic Paralysis Network Inc., (PPNI) has a forum containing three distinct discussion groups. We have an educational, support and advocacy discussion group; a discussion board to discuss our book, *living with Periodic Paralysis: The Mystery Unraveled,* and a discussion group for genealogy research looking for genetic-and genealogical connections among the members as a possible tool to be used in diagnosis. Our Facebook Group for educational discussion, support and advocacy with over 300 members, is used most frequently. The members prefer it to be a private board for obvious confidentiality reasons. There is a wide variety of information posted about many aspects of Periodic Paralysis. We interact in real time nearly every day with other members. We occasionally take polls and many members research and post scholarly and non-scholarly articles. We occasionally have web cam discussion groups and we continue to do research and provide the latest information to our members.

The PPNI works toward the improvement of the quality and safety of patients from all over the world with the various forms of Periodic Paralysis. Our focus is on educational resources to build self-reliance and self-empowerment and to prevent possible harm from improper treatment. Our approach to treatment focuses on the self-monitoring of an individuals vitals and the management of symptoms through natural methods. We also offer strategies to understanding the disease, getting a proper diagnosis, managing the symptoms, and assisting caregivers and family members. Due to these issues the Periodic Paralysis Network, Inc. is now considered to be a patient-safety-related organization or "advocacy" Group. We provide to our members: hope through education of all issues related to Periodic Paralysis, open and free discussion of thoughts and ideas, encouragement, support, sympathy, empathy, validation and now advocacy. We are now listed in the Advocate Directory at www.advocatedirectory.org.

In addition to joining a discussion group, everyone should also research Periodic Paralysis on the Internet. There are many Web sites with updated and quality information. Many other Web sites are not so careful about the accuracy of posted information and the reader should exercise caution before forming any conclusions about Periodic Paralysis. Most of the available research is difficult to read and understand. Some is very misleading, especially for those with unknown variants. Very little information exists on how to deal with the symptoms in a natural way, which is necessary for many people who have medication intolerances.

The Periodic Paralysis Network has a website and blog which contain a wide range of information. The Periodic Paralysis Network was created to provide a hands-on approach to understanding the disease, getting a proper diagnosis, managing the symptoms, and assisting caregivers and family members. We attempt to discuss issues relating to Periodic Paralysis in practical language. Our hope also is that the medical professionals dealing with individuals with Periodic Paralysis may come to our site and learn more about how to recognize, diagnose and properly treat their patients in a timely manner.

The third method for learning about Periodic Paralysis is by reading about it in books. However, only a few books exist with information about Periodic Paralysis and what is available is very specific to certain types or variants. They are also difficult to read and understand. Our book, *living with Periodic Paralysis: The Mystery Unraveled* was written in part for that reason and with that in mind. It is a culmination of all aspects of the condition in one book written in an easy to read format of narrative style, essays and technical input where necessary. It is also designed so the reader does not need to read from cover-to-cover, although that is a possibility, but rather a particular topic can be searched for and found easily for quick answers.

Notes

The following links belong to the Periodic Paralysis Forum:

Periodic Paralysis Network Website
http://www.periodicparalysisnetwork.com

Periodic Paralysis Support and Education Group
https://www.facebook.com/groups/periodicparalysisnetworksupportgroup/

Living With Periodic Paralysis: The Blog
http://livingwithperiodicparalysis.blogspot.com/

Periodic Paralysis Book Discussion Group
https://www.facebook.com/groups/periodicparalysisnetwork/

Periodic Paralysis Network Genealogy
https://www.facebook.com/groups/580168915344191/

Periodic Paralysis Network Page
https://www.facebook.com/PeriodicParalysisNetwork

Susan Q. Knittle-Hunter and Calvin Hunter Authors Page
https://www.facebook.com/SusanQKnittleHunterauthor

Periodic Paralysis Network Pinterest
www.pinterest.com/sqknittle/periodic-paralysis-network/

My favorite websites, groups, pages, and blogs related to Periodic Paralysis:

_____
_____
_____
_____
_____
_____
_____
_____
_____
_____
_____
_____
_____
_____
_____
_____
_____
_____
_____
_____

Notes

Eight
Describe Your Episodes
PARALYSIS – ACCOMPANYING SYMPTOMS

Know and Understand Your Symptoms
- Identify Paralytic Episodes
- Identify Other Symptoms
- Describe Episodes

Introduction

There are various ways in which the paralytic episodes can manifest themselves. Depending on the potassium levels; high, low or in normal ranges found in the blood serum levels, (to be discussed later), and the speed with which the potassium shifts, the episodes or attacks can be markedly different. Episodes may be as simple as dizziness, numbness or tingling, passing out, sudden dropping or falling to the ground or partial paralysis. They may be as serious as full body paralysis including heart arrhythmia, choking, the cessation of breathing and cardiac arrest. Attacks may happen as often as several a day or one or two in a lifetime. They may last from just a few minutes to hours at a time. Some individuals with known genetic markers for Periodic Paralysis may never go into paralysis.

Symptoms That Accompany the Paralytic Attacks

Some symptoms may over-lap so it is best to use a potassium reader (discussed later in the book), to measure the levels of potassium before treating, especially if one has Andersen-Tawil Syndrome or an ATS-like condition before treating based on the symptoms. If a potassium reader is not available, however, understanding what the symptoms indicate can very well help to know how to treat the episode.

Hypokalemic Periodic Paralysis

When potassium shifts into lower ranges in normal individuals, hypokalemia, low potassium levels in the blood, will occur for anyone and a myriad of symptoms can be experienced. Potassium regulates contractions of smooth muscles so when potassium is low muscle twitches, muscle spasms, charley horses and restless leg syndrome can occur. It plays a part in arranging the energy sources in the body so low levels of potassium can cause one to feel tired, fatigued and achy. It can also cause one to feel anxious, irritable and depressed. Potassium stops the destruction of bone, so when levels are low, osteoporosis can develop. Very low levels of potassium in the body can be dangerous, even deadly.

Symptoms typical of Hypokalemic Periodic Paralysis are found on page twenty-one.

Hyperkalemic Periodic Paralysis

When potassium shifts into higher ranges in normal individuals, hyperkalemia, high potassium levels in the blood, will occur for anyone and a myriad of symptoms can be experienced and can be dangerous, even deadly. If an individual has Hyperkalemic Periodic Paralysis and potassium shifts into higher ranges, he or she can and will experience a combination of the same myriad of symptoms as well as paralysis and can be equally as dangerous and deadly.

Symptoms typical of Hyperkalemic Periodic Paralysis are found on page twenty-two.

Andersen-Tawil Syndrome

An individual with Andersen-Tawil Syndrome may experience the symptoms described previously depending on whether the potassium shifts into high or low ranges. The symptoms will be based on the triggers and will coincide with hypokalemia, hyperkalemia or normokalemia as described previously. They also experience long QT interval heartbeats (which is a marker for Andersen-Tawil Syndrome), a life threatening arrhythmia in which the heart takes longer than it should to recharge and they have ventricular arrhythmia and which is a marker for ATS. That is a problem originating in the lower chambers of the heart. They include premature ventricular contractions known as PVC's; bigeminy, trigeminy, and quadrigeminy beats in which PVC's occur every second, third or fourth beat; ventricular tachycardia in which there are at least three PVC's in a row and ventricular fibrillation a beat without any organized contraction which is life threatening. Fainting, called syncope, is common.

More symptoms typical of Andersen-Tawil Syndrome are found on page twenty-four.

Normokalemic Periodic Paralysis

For some individuals, periodic episodes of paralysis may occur when potassium shifts within normal ranges. This is called Normokalemic Periodic Paralysis. Some studies indicate that it is actually a variant of Hyperkalemic Periodic Paralysis. It should also be noted here that paralyzed muscles swell and fill with potassium. When the swelling begins to subside the level of potassium may return to normal levels. This may happen quickly and by the time the blood sample is taken the level of potassium may have already returned to the normal ranges, thus appearing to be Normokalemia.

If someone has this condition or appears to have it, when this happens he or she can and will experience a combination of the same myriad of symptoms either Hypokalemic Periodic Paralysis or Hyperkalemic Periodic Paralysis. Normokalemic Periodic Paralysis can be seen in individuals with Andersen-Tawil Syndrome.

Paramyotonia Congenita

One who suffers with Paramyotonia Congenita may experience a variety of symptoms, but usually the skeletal muscles can become stiff, tight, and tense or they can become contracted and weak. Due to the fact that PMC is actually considered to be a form of

Describe Your Episodes

Hyperkalemic Periodic Paralysis, the symptoms will be the same as seen in Hyperkalemic Periodic Paralysis.

Thyrotoxic Periodic Paralysis

An individual with Thyrotoxic Periodic Paralysis typically suffers with symptoms exactly like Hypokalemic Periodic Paralysis. They also have high levels of the thyroid hormone.

Abortive Attacks

Abortive attacks are periods of extended time anywhere from hours, days, weeks or months in which some individuals are totally debilitated by extreme muscle weakness without going into full paralysis. The previously described common symptoms may begin but the full attack or total paralysis may not occur. The person is left with severe weakness and other symptoms such as extreme fatigue. It is difficult to do anything physically and it also can affect cognition abilities, such as memory, thought processing and speech and some become very fragile emotionally. The individual may want to sleep and may have no appetite. In my own case the abortive attacks are totally debilitating and actually worse than the episodes of paralysis. When I am in them, I wish I could slip into paralysis and get it "over with." I have experienced no worse feelings of weakness and helplessness in my life other than being in a full body state of paralysis.

Many people attempt to 'push through' abortive attacks, but actually more muscle damage can occur from exertion during these episodes than from the paralytic attacks. It is essential to remain resting and calm until the attack has passed.

Other Types of Periodic Paralysis Episodes

Although distinct episodes of total, full body paralysis are a clear sign of Periodic Paralysis, it must be noted here that not every paralytic episode is full body or total paralysis. An individual may be only partially paralyzed. Only his or her legs may be paralyzed or they may only be weak. Episodes may occur as sudden falls or dropping to the floor. Feet or legs or arms may go numb and tingly. Muscles in the calves may become very tight and painful. An episode may include overall weakness with arrhythmias and fluctuating blood pressure. Walking may suddenly become difficult due to a weak foot.

Each of these attacks or episodes has a clear beginning and a clear end. Each episode is intermittent. They come and go. Most people will be normal between them or their muscle strength will improve between them. However, some individuals over time may develop permanent muscle weakness.

Description of an Episode

The following is my description of what it is like being in a full-body, total, paralytic episode. It was written at a time when I still did not know what was happening to me.

> *"Usually, I wake up in the morning and I am paralyzed. I find I can't move. I can't open my eyes. My mouth is open. I cannot breathe*

through my nose. I have urges to swallow but cannot so there is a choking sound in my throat every few minutes. Sometimes my heart will race or beat irregularly, though usually, there is no problem with my heart. My mouth is very dry. I cannot speak

As I begin to come out of it, my mouth will start to get saliva, my eyes will open but I can only see what is in front of me, since I cannot move my head. Sometimes my eyes will jerk around when I first open them, usually jerking up. My body will sometimes jerk a little. Sometimes there is a big breath my body will take.

Sometimes, I will go back into it. My eyes close, I feel very hot and all the symptoms return. Sometimes there will be a few jerks as I go back into it.

During all of this I am awake and am aware of everything going on around me. Sometimes I begin to cry, due to the frustration, and fear. I can feel the tears running down my cheeks.

If I have these at times other than upon waking, the symptoms are the same. I get a strange sensation of heat body wide, usually beginning in my back. My eyes will close and then my body goes limp. I may have a few jerks as I am going limp. My mouth will open and I am in it…unable to move, speak or open my eyes.

Sometimes, I do not go too deep. It is all the same but I am able to open my eyes and can speak a little with a tight tongue and tight lips. My mouth is still open, however. I cannot move my body.

Once one of these begins, it may last up to 45 minutes to an hour, or can be as short as about ten minutes, if it is a second or third one in a row.

It takes about fifteen to thirty minutes to come out of it all the way. I am always left with lingering weakness for many hours that can linger into days. Speaking is difficult. Walking is difficult. My arms and hands come back sooner than my legs. I begin to get feeling back in my body. I can move my lips. I begin to breath thru my nose again. It is difficult to speak or move but it gradually comes back. Speech is very difficult; my lips do not want to move. My tongue is difficult to move. I will suddenly have an urgency to urinate. If, at this point, I get help to the bathroom, I am like a rag doll, especially my legs. My arms flail, like a child just learning to stand and walk; balancing herself.

For many hours, I remain too weak to do much of anything but sit up in bed or sit in a recliner. I must use my walker or a wheelchair.

It is difficult to know what brings these episodes on. I know that sleep

Describe Your Episodes

> *has something to do with some of them, but not all of them. I know that sometimes, when I wake up during the night with an urgency to urinate, I am coming out of one, because I have all of the symptoms previously discussed. My arms and hands and legs are numb and feeling is just coming back. My mouth is tight and dry. Walking is difficult." (May 28, 2010)*

Describe your own symptoms and paralytic episodes in Chapter Twelve.

Notes _____
_____
_____
_____
_____
_____
_____
_____
_____
_____
_____
_____
_____
_____
_____
_____
_____
_____
_____
_____
_____
_____
_____
_____
_____
_____
_____
_____
_____
_____
_____
_____
_____
_____
_____
_____

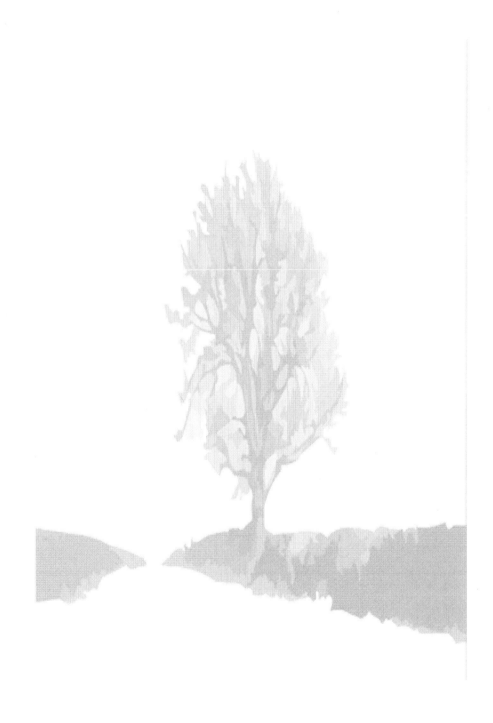

Nine
Monitor Your Vitals
TOOLS FOR THE JOB

- ❖ **Monitor your vitals**
  - ➤ **Obtain medical equipment**
    - **Potassium reader**
    - **Oximeter**
    - **Stethoscope**
    - **Wrist blood pressure device**
    - **Ear thermometer**
    - **PH monitor**
    - **Blood sugar monitor**

Introduction

Having several medical devices gathered for use during paralytic episodes is an important issue for individuals with Periodic Paralysis, their family members and/or caregivers. It is essential to have everything ready when needed. Taking the "guessing" or the "unknown" out of the equation makes a very big difference for everyone concerned.

As previously discussed, Periodic Paralysis is a very rare mineral metabolic disorder. Individuals with various forms of PP suffer the effects of partial or full body muscle weakness or paralysis, which may be accompanied by very serious symptoms. On a cellular level, triggered by things such as sleep, exercise, sugar, salt, most medications, stress, cold, heat, anesthesia, adrenaline, IVs, etc., potassium wrongly enters the muscles either temporarily weakening or paralyzing the individual. Episodes can be full body lasting hours or days. Dangerous heart arrhythmia, heart rate fluctuation, blood pressure fluctuation, choking, breathing difficulties, cardiac arrest and/or respiratory arrest can also accompany the episodes. Due to these complications, it is extremely important to monitor the vitals of the individual during an episode.

Monitoring your vital signs diligently is the most important way to manage the serious complications. Most people in full body paralysis are unable to describe how they are feeling or what is happening to them, so there is only one way for sure to know how the body is functioning; using medical devices to measure things such as oxygen level, body temperature, blood pressure, heart and breathing rates, potassium levels, pH levels and blood sugar levels. If someone can describe how they are feeling, it is still impossible to know what is going on inside the body on a cellular level. It can be unsafe to make decisions about interventions without the correct information. Guessing about the intervention could trigger serious and/or life-threatening conditions. Avoiding calling for an ambulance every time a paralytic episode occurs, is another benefit to being prepared with a collection of medical devices for measuring vital signs. Going to the hospital is stressful, expensive and unnecessary in most cases, as well as possibly life-threatening if the medical professionals are not familiar with Periodic Paralysis.

We discovered that several pieces of medical equipment could be very handy for measuring your vitals. These include: a potassium meter, a finger pulse oximeter, blood sugar monitor, stethoscope, wrist blood pressure monitor, a thermometer and a digital pH balance reader. These items are necessary for caregivers to monitor vitals primarily because the person in paralysis is usually unable to communicate. The vitals serve as the communication tool. Keeping written records is very important especially when making connections between individual events. The same holds true for the measurement and recording of other vitals such as blood pressure, temperature, blood sugar levels, oxygen levels, respiration, heart rate and the input and output of fluids.

We purchased all of these devices and Calvin was able to know what was happening when I was in paralysis and he was able to make decisions about how to treat my symptoms or if he should call for an ambulance. He recorded the information to later share with the doctors. There are charts for recording the data below.

Potassium Reader

There are two types of potassium readers, however, one has been discontinued. Neither one is a medical device. This means medical insurance will not pay for them and they are very expensive. The newest one is easier to use but costs about $350.00. It measures the potassium level in either the blood or the saliva. Using one of these little devices will give one a baseline for their normal levels and for when their potassium is high or low. We now know that most of us who have various forms of Periodic Paralysis have our own level of normal and our own unique level of what is high or low for us as an individual. Keeping record of our findings is very important. Although not recognized by many doctors, some are willing to recognize their worth and rely on the findings. During an episode, one's potassium levels can be checked as often as possible or needed. Caregivers can decide how to proceed if the levels are too high or too low.

Normal potassium levels range from 3.5 to 5.0 mEq/L however; "normal" potassium levels among individuals with PP can be different than this norm. It is extremely important to discover what is "normal" for each person in order to know when the levels may be high or low. Using a potassium meter is the best way to discover that level or what is called a "baseline." If an individual cannot afford to purchase one of these devices, symptoms can indicate high or low potassium levels. There are lists of symptoms, which typically accompany different levels of potassium in Chapters Four and Six for reference.[1]

The following videos demonstrate how to use a cardy meter.

Video: Cardy Meter Potassium Test:
https://www.youtube.com/watch?v=jB3pJCFRil8&list=FLOap26pdr8A_Ze2gt3rv8Mg&index=25

Video: Cardy Meter Calibration
https://www.youtube.com/watch?v=_S-roOpSTC0&list=FLOap26pdr8A_Ze2gt3rv8Mg&index=24

Monitor Your Vitals

Digital Oximeter

The digital oximeter is a small and inexpensive device, which reads the oxygen level in our blood. It is placed on the tip of a finger to get the reading. This reading is important, because when in paralysis, our oxygen levels may drop. If oxygen levels dip too low and oxygen is not handy, it can indicate that an ambulance may need to be called due to hypoxemia, which is low oxygen in the blood. The device also displays the heart rate and intensity. The caregivers will know if the patient is in tachycardia (fast) or bradycardia (slow) heart rate and arrhythmia (irregular heart beat).

Normal Oxygen =100% to 95%
Low Oxygen = < 90% Hypoxemia[1]
Compromise of organs = < 80% [2]

Normal Heart Rate: resting = 60 to 100 bpm
Too Fast Heart Rate: Tachycardia = > 100 bpm
Too Slow Heart Rate: Bradycardia = < 60 bpm [7]

pH Meter or pH Strips

Because Periodic Paralysis is a mineral metabolic disorder, individuals with PP are prone to developing metabolic acidosis (too much acidity) or metabolic alkalosis (too much alkalinity) in their body. These are serious conditions and can be life threatening. This device measures for pH imbalance in the urine, saliva or blood. Paper strips are also available and very easy to use as well as reasonable priced. PH levels:

Blood pH levels: Acidosis= 1 to 7.40　Neutral= 7.41　Alkalosis= 7.42 to 14.0
Urine pH levels:　Not healthy < 6　　Neutral 6.5 to 8.0　Not healthy > 8.5
Saliva pH levels: Not healthy < 6.5　　Neutral= 6.6 to 6.7　Not healthy > 6.8 [3]

More Information about metabolic acidosis can be found at:
http://livingwithperiodicparalysis.blogspot.com/2013/12/periodic-paralysis-and-metabolic.html

Blood Sugar/Glucose Monitor

These devices are readily available. Though used normally for individuals with diabetes or hypoglycemia, the meters are important devices for those with PP. Having high sugar levels may trigger an episode. When the body stresses during an episode, sugar levels may rise. If the sugar moves with the potassium, it may cause pain in the muscles. The finger-stick device for pricking the finger may also be used with the potassium reader. The strips are very expensive. If a doctor prescribes them, they are usually paid for by insurance.

Normal fasting blood sugar 70 to 100 mg/dL
Normal blood sugar two hours after eating < 140 mg/dL
Normal not fasting < 125 mg/dL
Before a meal 90 to 130 mg/dL
After a meal < 180 mg/dL [4]

Wrist Blood Pressure Cuff

Knowing the patients blood pressure is extremely important. The levels may get dangerously low or high and indicate the need for an ambulance. These devices also display the heart rate and arrhythmia. Having it on the wrist is so much easier than trying to use the older methods and tools for measuring blood pressure, during an episode.

Low blood pressure < 90/60
Normal blood pressure   90/60 to 120/80
Borderline blood pressure 120/80 to 140/90

High blood pressure > 140/90
Emergency > 180/110 [5]

Digital Thermometer

The digital thermometer, which can be used in the ear, is a good choice. It is easy and quick to use by a caregiver when an individual is in paralysis. If someone with PP has an infection in his or her body, this can trigger an episode. This information may be useful to the caregiver. 98.6 is typically normal, but each person has an individual "normal" that can be higher or lower. Getting a baseline for the individual is important.[6]

Stethoscope

Due to the serious nature of irregular heartbeats, a stethoscope can be an important tool to have handy. If the wrist blood pressure cuff or the digital oximeter indicates irregular heartbeats, fast heartbeats or slow heartbeats the caregiver can then listen to try to detect them and decide how serious they may be. YouTube has many videos that teach how to understand the sounds of the heart.

With all of the tools in place and diligently recording the results, there is no more guessing. The caregivers are informed and can easily relax knowing precisely what is happening. As they take the measurements and record the results, they can tell the patient exactly what is happening. The patient can then relax, knowing they are out of danger. If, on the other hand, the results indicate an emergency situation, an ambulance can be called or the caregiver will know what to do and the patient will know that help is on the way. In conclusion, taking the "guessing" or the "unknown" out of the equation makes a very big difference for everyone concerned.

Without an oximeter, wrist blood pressure cuff or stethoscope, heart rate can be felt and measured by placing the tips of the first and second fingers on the wrist, the side of the neck, the top of a foot or inside an elbow. [7] Many websites exist which can describe how to do this and what to feel for and listen to, in order to detect a problem.

More information about the tools and where to purchase them can be found on the Periodic Paralysis Network Website:
http://www.periodicparalysisnetwork.com/toolssupplies.htm

Video: Medical Tool Kit For Monitoring Vitals:
https://www.youtube.com/watch?v=zqbcovGVHKw&index=26&list=FLOap26pdr8A_Ze2gt3rv8Mg

Monitor Your Vitals

In the fields of special education and medicine, it is said, "If it is not written down, it did not happen." We must document as much as we can for discovering our triggers, getting

a diagnosis, getting proper treatment, sharing with our medical professionals and more. Therefore, we have included several types of charts on the following pages to help you record every detail that we think is important. Some are blank for you to copy and others are completed to demonstrate how to use them.

Notes _____
_____
_____
_____
_____
_____
_____
_____
_____
_____
_____
_____
_____
_____
_____
_____
_____
_____
_____
_____
_____
_____
_____

Works Cited Chapter Five:
1. Wikipedia. (June 2014). Hypokalemia. Retrieved from:
http://en.wikipedia.org/wiki/Hypokalemia

2. Wikipedia. (June 2014). Oxygen saturation in medicine. Retrieved from:
http://en.wikipedia.org/wiki/Oxygen_saturation_in_medicine

3. Wikipedia. (June 2014). PH. Retrieved from:
http://en.wikipedia.org/wiki/PH

4. Wikipedia. (June 2014). Blood sugar. Retrieved from:
http://en.wikipedia.org/wiki/Blood_sugar

5. Wikipedia. (June 2014). Blood Pressure. Retrieved from:
http://en.wikipedia.org/wiki/Blood_pressure

6. Wikipedia. (June 2014). Human body temperature. Retrieved from:
http://en.wikipedia.org/wiki/Human_body_temperature

7. Wikipedia. (July 2014). Heart Rate. Retrieved from:
http://en.wikipedia.org/wiki/Heart_rate

Daily Potassium Measurement and Vitals Chart

Name **Date**
Top Line- Time   **Left Column-** Potassium Level   **Bottom-** Notes/Other Levels

	am						pm									
	6	7	8	9	10	11	12	1	2	3	4	5	6	7	8	9	10
0																	
1																	
2																	
3																	
4																	
5																	
6																	
7																	
8																	

6	7	8	9	10	11	12	1	2	3	4	5	6	7	8	9	10

Notes/Activity/ Symptoms/ Blood Pressure/ Heart Rate/ Arrhythmia/ Oxygen/ pH level/ Temperature/ Sugar

Periodic Paralysis Network   Sequim, Washington U.S.A. All rights reserved. Copyright © 2014

Monitor Your Vitals

Daily Potassium Measurement and Vitals Chart

Name Susan **Date** 10-30-10
Top Line- Time **Left Column-** Potassium Level **Bottom-** Notes/Other Levels

Notes/Activity/ Symptoms/ Blood Pressure/ Heart Rate/ Arrhythmia/ Oxygen/ pH level/ Temperature/ Sugar
Periodic Paralysis Network Sequim, Washington U.S.A. All rights reserved. Copyright © 2014

This is a completed chart with information taken from when I was really struggling from the effects of two antibiotics. We did not know why at the time. At the time we did not have a wrist blood pressure cuff so blood pressure readings are not added. The plots in the top of the chart give a good graph to easily see where the potassium levels increased into the 7.5 ranges. This can be very useful in attempting to get a diagnosis or finding a trigger. This proved my problem with two separate antibiotics and the next day, which was worse, coupled with a heart Holter monitor proved my long QT at the same time as my paralytic episodes.

Daily Potassium Measurement Chart

Name   **Date**

	am											pm												
	1	2	3	4	5	6	7	8	9	10	11	12	1	2	3	4	5	6	7	8	9	10	11	12
1																								
1.2																								
1.4																								
1.6																								
1.8																								
2.0																								
2.2																								
2.4																								
2.6																								
2.8																								
3.0																								
3.2																								
3.4																								
3.6																								
3.8																								
4.0																								
4.2																								
4.4																								
4.6																								
4.8																								
5.0																								
5.2																								
5.4																								
5.6																								
5.8																								
6.0																								
6.2																								
6.4																								
6.6																								
6.8																								
7.0																								
7.2																								
7.4																								
7.6																								
7.8																								
8.0																								

Place a dot or x in the box or on the line (.1, .3, .5, .7, .9) then connect dots for graph.

Periodic Paralysis Network Sequim, Washington U.S.A. All rights reserved. Copyright © 2014

Monitor Your Vitals

Daily Potassium Measurement Chart

Place a dot or x in the box or on the line (.1, .3, .5, .7, .9) then connect dots for graph.
Periodic Paralysis Network Sequim, Washington U.S.A. All rights reserved. Copyright © 2014

The Daily Potassium Measurement Chart is designed to chart only the daily potassium levels. It records 24 hours. The time is across the top and the potassium levels are in the left column. The results of the potassium meter can easily be plotted. The even numbers (.2, .4, .6, .8, .0) are plotted in the box with an x or a dot. The odd numbers (.1, .3, .5, .7, .9) are plotted on the lines with an x or a dot. The x's or dots can be connected to form a graph. The normal potassium levels are found in the center of the chart between the shaded rows. This is to easily see the high or low shifts.

The Periodic Paralysis Guide And Workbook

Date	1	2	3	4	5	6	Date	1	2	3	4	5	6
Time							Time						
Sleep							Sleep						
Potassium							Potassium						
Glucose							Glucose						
pH Level							pH Level						
Temp							Temp						
B/P							B/P						
Heart							Heart						
Arrhyth							Arrhyth						
Oxygen							Oxygen						

Date	1	2	3	4	5	6	Date	1	2	3	4	5	6
Time							Time						
Sleep							Sleep						
Potassium							Potassium						
Glucose							Glucose						
pH Level							pH Level						
Temp							Temp						
B/P							B/P						
Heart							Heart						
Arrhyth							Arrhyth						
Oxygen							Oxygen						

Daily Vitals Chart

Comments:

Periodic Paralysis Network Sequim, Washington U.S.A. All rights reserved. Copyright © 2014

Monitor Your Vitals

Date 6-30	1	2	3	4	5	6
Time	6:00					
Sleep	8					
Potassium	4.3					
Glucose	99					
pH Level	7.2					
Temp	97.3					
B/P						
Heart	63					
Arrhyth	No					
Oxygen	94					

Date 7-1	1	2	3	4	5	6
Time	6:15					
Sleep	5.5					
Potassium	3.4					
Glucose	101					
pH Level	7.0					
Temp	98.1					
B/P						
Heart	60					
Arrhyth						
Oxygen	92					

Date	1	2	3	4	5	6
Time						
Sleep						
Potassium						
Glucose						
pH Level						
Temp						
B/P						
Heart						
Arrhyth						
Oxygen						

Date	1	2	3	4	5	6
Time						
Sleep						
Potassium						
Glucose						
pH Level						
Temp						
B/P						
Heart						
Arrhyth						
Oxygen						

Date	1	2	3	4	5	6
Time						
Sleep						
Potassium						
Glucose						
pH Level						
Temp						
B/P						
Heart						
Arrhyth						
Oxygen						

Daily Vitals Chart Susan

Comments: 6-30 Paralysis during the night. 7-1 Prepare lists, low on night.

This weekly Daily Vitals Chart is designed to easily record a full week of recordings and to easily spot abnormalities and progress. There are six time slots for each day and a list of the important vitals needed to track. There is a section for comments.

Notes

Ten
Identify And Eliminate Triggers
AVOID - CHART - JOURNAL - MONITOR

❖ **Identify and eliminate all known triggers**
  ➢ Record symptoms and possible causes
  ➢ Monitor symptoms
  ➢ Keep a journal

Introduction

This chapter will discuss the elements or experiences, which trigger or activate the potassium to shift causing the attacks of periodic paralysis and how to identify them. There are some common triggers among those with the different forms of Periodic Paralysis and there are some triggers, which are unique for each individual. Triggers can be certain medications, foods, activities, stress or even sleep. It is important to know one's triggers in order to avoid having episodes or attacks of paralysis due to permanent damage, which may occur to organs in the body.

One of the most important things a person with Periodic Paralysis can do, no matter which type they have, is to discover what causes, starts or triggers our episodes of muscle weakness or paralysis. There are many triggers that set into motion the partial and total paralysis and other symptoms. It is important to discover these triggers because we need to stop the episodes or attacks, if possible, in order to regain the quality of our lives and to prevent the damage being done to our organs as the potassium shifts and depletes or increases in our bodies.

Potassium shifting can cause a myriad of conditions and the symptoms that accompany them, as discussed previously, including permanent tightness of the calf muscles or muscle wasting of arm and leg muscles, restless leg syndrome or even osteoporosis. The breathing and swallowing muscles can weaken over time and be affected during attacks. If this happens it is an extremely serious and emergency situation. Dangerous arrhythmias of the heart can also occur when an individual is in an episode or attack. In the case of people with Andersen-Tawil Syndrome, the paralysis leads to tachycardia and serious arrhythmia, including long QT intervals, which can lead to cardiac arrest. Other complications can include respiratory arrest causing death or aspiration pneumonia after an attack, causing death. Though rare, these can occur with Hypokalemic Periodic Paralysis. Complications of Hyperkalemic Periodic Paralysis include bi-directional heart arrhythmias causing sudden death and permanent weakness of the muscles. Between attacks, the muscles usually return to normal or strengthen, but over time with repeated episodes of paralysis, progressive and permanent weakness of the muscles which can be severe is possible. This includes the heart and breathing muscles. This can lead to heart failure and respiratory failure, thus eventual death. Avoiding paralysis is absolutely necessary, due to these life-threatening effects.

The Periodic Paralysis Guide And Workbook

The easiest way to decide what caused an episode or symptoms would be to look at anything new or different; a new type of bread, a new antibiotic, a new activity, a new shampoo, stressful event (good or bad), or a chilled or over heated room. Discovering our triggers requires a little bit of time to follow a simple plan. In a matter of a few days or weeks, it may be possible to draw some useful conclusions about the possible triggers of a paralytic event and the symptom, which can accompany them.

In the fields of medicine and education, it is said, "If you did not write it down, it did not happen." This can be applied to our method for discovering our triggers. The first thing we must do is to write everything down. Creating a journal is a good way to make sure this is done. I have created a chart, which can be added to a journal to make the process easier (see a copy below).

Several necessary components are included on this chart:

- A 24-hour time frame
- A section to write possible triggers
- A section to write down symptoms and vitals one may be experiencing
- A section to record the muscle weakness and paralysis
- This section becomes a graph of the periods of weakness or paralysis

Once the information has been gathered for a few weeks, it will be easy to see trends or connections of a particular food, medication or activity to muscle weakness or paralysis.

The following are lists of the common possible symptoms of Periodic Paralysis one may experience as well as the paralysis and muscle weakness and the triggers, which may set them into motion.

Understanding and becoming familiar with the symptoms is another important part of completing the chart. As much information that can be added will be helpful. In this section anything may be included from "**feeling well**," or "**none**," to some of the known symptoms for hyperkalemia and hypokalemia in the following charts.

Notes_____
_____
_____
_____
_____
_____
_____
_____
_____
_____
_____
_____
_____

Identify And Eliminate Triggers

Notes

The Periodic Paralysis Guide And Workbook

The following are at-a-glance lists of typical symptoms for the different forms of Periodic Paralysis. For more symptoms refer to Chapter Four.

The Symptoms Typical Of Low Potassium:

- Episodic muscle weakness
- Episodic partial paralysis
- Episodic total paralysis
- Episodic flaccid paralysis (limp muscles, without tone)
- Muscle weakness after exercise
- Muscle weakness
- Muscle stiffness
- Muscle aches
- Muscle cramps
- Muscle contractions
- Muscle spasms
- Muscle tenderness
- Pins and needles sensation
- Eyelid myotonia (cannot open eyelid after opening and then closing them)
- Irritability
- Severe thirst
- Abdominal bloating
- Nausea
- Vomiting
- Constipation
- Excessive urination
- Sweating
- Tachycardia
- Irregular heartbeat
- Palpatations
- Dizziness
- Fainting
- Breathing problems (barely breathing)
- Hypoventilation
- Increase in blood pressure
- Irritability

Vitals To Add To The Chart As Symptoms:

- Potassium level
- pH level (saliva)
- pH level (urine)
- Glucose (sugar) level
- Temperature
- Blood pressure
- Heart rate
- Arrhythmia
- Oxygen

Identify And Eliminate Triggers

The Symptoms Typical Of High Potassium:

- Episodic muscle weakness
- Episodic partial paralysis
- Episodic total paralysis
- Muscle contraction or rigidity during an attack
- Muscle weakness
- Muscle cramps
- Muscle stiffness
- Fasciculation (muscle twitching)
- Pins and needles sensation
- Cramping pain
- Reduced reflexes
- Muscle contraction involving tongue
- Slurring of words
- Tightness in legs
- Strange feeling in legs
- Tingling sensations
- Pulse issues (absent, slow, or weak)
- Irregular heart beat
- Heart palpitations
- Breathing problems (wheezing, shortness of breath, fast breathing)
- Mild hyperventilation
- Decrease in blood pressure
- Nausea
- Feeling hot
- Sleepiness

More Possible Symptoms For The Chart:

- Headache
- Chest pain
- Numbness
- Unable to walk
- Agitation
- Shallow breathing
- Pain in calves
- Cramps in legs
- Restless legs
- Burning in feet
- Hyperventilation
- Feeling cold
- Clammy
- Dizzy
- Shaky
- Unsteady
- Rubbery legs
- Hunger
- Jerking
- Awake
- Confusion
- Strange feeling in legs
- Brain fog
- Sleeplessness
- Memory problem
- Depression
- Weakness
- Constipation
- Foot drop
- Dry mouth
- Choking
- Angry

Triggers

The Common Triggers Of Hypokalemic Periodic Paralysis

The triggers usually responsible for causing potassium to shift in Hypokalemic Periodic Paralysis are:

- Eating a large amount of carbohydrates in a meal
- Drinking alcohol
- Ingesting too much salt
- Stress (good or bad)
- Excitement
- Fear
- Vigorous exercise
- Resting after exercise
- Cold
- Epinephrine/adrenaline
- Cold
- Anesthesia

The Common Triggers Of Hyperkalemic Periodic Paralysis

The triggers usually responsible for causing potassium to shift in Hyperkalemic Periodic Paralysis are:

- Eating a large amount of carbohydrates in a meal
- Exercise
- Cold
- Ingesting too much potassium in food or medications
- Stress (good or bad)
- Rest after exercise
- Fatigue
- Fasting
- Cigarette smoke

The Common Triggers Of Paramyotonia Congenita

The triggers usually responsible for causing potassium to shift in Paramyotonia Congenita are:
- Exercise
- Exertion
- Repetitious movement
- Cold
- Sleeping in

Identify And Eliminate Triggers

Other Triggers For Periodic Paralysis

Triggers can include:

Diet: Diet can be one of the biggest contributors to episodes of paralysis. The following are some of my offenders or those that have been reported to me or I have found in the research:
- Simple carbohydrates: sugar, white flour and more
- Complex carbohydrates: some grains, wheat, rye and more
- Meat: mostly red meats
- Salt
- Caffeine
- MSG
- Alcohol
- Large meals
- Gluten

Sleep:
All aspects of sleep may set episodes into motion:
- Falling asleep
- During sleep
- Waking up

Other:
- Dehydration
- Fasting
- Sitting too long
- Changes in the weather
- Fatigue
- Heat
- Cold
- Electromagnetic Force (EMF's)
- Menstrual cycle

Exercise:
Some individuals have no problem with exercise but others may not be able to tolerate any type of exercise or very little exercise. This is called "exercise intolerance." Episodes may develop soon after or the next day.
Rest after exercise: may set an episode into motion.

Unknown: One can follow all the rules and still have episodes for unknown reasons.

Over-the-counter medications:
Most over the counter medications, can set muscle weakness or paralysis into motion for people with Periodic Paralysis. The following is a list of some known offenders.
- Cough syrups
- Eye drops
- Glycerin enemas
- NSAID's

Compounds or Chemicals:
If the following ingredients are in any products you use...you should stop using them until you are sure they are not causing symptoms:
- Sodium Hydroxide
- Edetate Disodium
- Stearic Acid

They may be in any of the following:
Lotions, oils, hair dyes or colors, antiperspirants, enemas, suppositories, soaps, shampoos, shaving creams, foams, toothpastes, deodorants, beauty products, skincare products, cosmetic products, bath salts, emollients, ointments, creams, hair sprays, perfumes, colognes, powders, hair gels, oils, tonics, mousse

Drugs:
Many, many drugs can set muscle weakness or paralysis into motion for people with Periodic Paralysis.

If one must take a drug, it is better to begin with ¼ of a normal dose to make sure it will work for you.

- Saline drips, glucose Infusion: If an IV is needed, mannitol can be used
(or diluted solutions in extreme cases)
- Oral or Intravenous Corticosteroids
- Muscle relaxers
- Beta blockers
- Tranquilizers
- Pain killers (analgesics)
- Antihistamines
- Puffers for asthma
- Antibiotics
- Cough syrups
- Eye drops to dilate eyes
- Contrast dye for MRI's
- Lidocaine
- Anesthetics
- Epinepherine (Can sometimes help symptoms of Hyperkalemic Periodic Paralysis)
- Adrenaline (Can sometimes help symptoms of Hyperkalemic Periodic Paralysis)

For more information about the medications or drugs which can cause muscle weakness, muscle paralysis, long QT interval hearts beats (ATS) and torsades de pointes (ATS), please go to:

http://www.periodicparalysisnetwork.com/pdf/What%20are%20the%20Periodic%20Paralysis%20Triggers.pdf

Identify And Eliminate Triggers

Notes

Trigger Chart

Date	6am	7am	8am	9am	10am	11am	12pm	1pm	2pm	3pm	4pm	5pm	6pm	7pm	8pm	9pm	10pm	11pm	12am	1am	2am	3am	4am	5am
Food, Drink, Meds, Activity																								
Symptoms																								

Conditions	Total Paralysis	Partial Paralysis	Total Weakness	Partial Weakness	Numbness	Normal

Identify And Eliminate Triggers

Completing the Trigger Chart:

- ❖ Fill in the date.
- ❖ Begin recording your activities, food, drink and medications in the top section. Start at the time you wake up. Include all food eaten in a meal. Record what you are doing, for instance sitting, eating, reading, exercising, walking, cooking, shopping or more.
- ❖ Record how you are feeling, for instance, good, very thirsty, constipated, confusion, sleepy, unsteady, legs are weak, total paralysis or more.
- ❖ Put a check mark in, (or fill in) the box that best describes your condition, for instance normal, weak, more weak, partial paralysis, more partial paralysis, or total paralysis.
- ❖ Continue this through your day, it is not necessary to do it at night, but you may want to include paralysis, numbness, or more, if it is happening at night.
- ❖ The bottom of the chart will become a graph and it will aid in seeing the times of symptoms.

In the completed chart below, we can see that two and one half to three hours after eating breakfast and taking septra, an antibiotic and a calcium tablet, the patient begins to experience weakness and then paralysis. It is a good chance that the medication or something eaten at breakfast was the cause.

If this person eats the same thing everyday and takes the calcium every morning, and the only new thing is the septra it would be safe to assume the antibiotic caused the episode. By four pm the episode has stopped. At five pm muscle weakness begins after an hour of being up and preparing dinner. This may be from exercise intolerance or due to something eaten at lunch.

If someone eats the same lunch everyday but does not always help with dinner, it could be safe to assume the exercise caused the weakness. The same could be true in reverse. At seven pm, overall weakness takes hold for the remainder of the evening. This may be from the food eaten at dinner or a continuation of the weakness from the earlier activity. During the night there are three episodes of total paralysis. Since sleep is a trigger, it may be impossible to stop the episodes throughout the night.

Trigger Chart

Date	Food, Drink, Meds, Activity	Symptoms	Conditions	Total Paralysis	Partial Paralysis	Total Weakness	Partial Weakness	Numbness	Normal
6am	Awake, Get up, Bathroom, Shower, Dress	Legs weak					■		
7am	Breakfast: Sugar milk, 8 Granicereal, egg, almonds, Take softw, Calcium Tablet	Fingers & below knees					■		
8am	Make Bed, Clean Kitchen	None							■
9am	In Recliner on Computer	None							■
10am	" "	Feet tired, weak, hot					■		
11am	" "	Slurring words, Legs Burn Cramping, Top paralyzed			■				
12pm	" "	Total Paralysis (can't open ears, breathe)	■						
1pm	Get Help to Bathroom, back to recliner	Eyes open to space, sudden improvement			■				
2pm	Eat Lunch in recliner Cheese, jicama, nuts, prunes	Less weak, hungry, Getting better					■		
3pm	Sit in recliner, Read	Still weak and tired					■		
4pm	Sit in recliner, Computer, Bathroom	Tired					■		
5pm	Help + TV dinner	None							■
6pm	Eat Dinner 1/2 Chicken Breast, Salad, Asparagus	None							■
7pm	Sit in recliner, Watch TV, Knit	Overall weakness					■		
8pm	Take m: ropey w/ butter milk " "	Overall weakness					■		
9pm	Bathroom, Get PJs on	Overall weakness, Tired					■		
10pm	Sleeping								
11pm									
12am									
1am	Wakes up	paralyzed		■					
2am	Sleep								
3am	Wakes up	paralyzed		■					
4am	Sleep								
5am	Wakes up	paralyzed		■					

Identify And Eliminate Triggers

Evaluating the Data

When looking at your completed charts, it is best to first check the periods of paralysis. Then check the activity, medications taken or food eaten two to three hours before that time. Was anything new? Was any activity out of the ordinary?

- ❖ Check period of paralysis or weakness:
  - ➢ Check two to three hours before.
    - ▪ New medication?
- ❖ New food, drink?
  - ➢ New activity?
    - ▪ More than usual?
    - ▪ Longer than usual?
- ❖ If answer is not clear: Continue to chart for a few days. If there seems to be a pattern:
  - ➢ Change only one thing at that time:
    - ▪ Remove sugar or
    - ▪ Cut medication dose or
  - ➢ Stop or reduce the activity
    - ▪ Less than usual
    - ▪ Shorter than usual
- ❖ Check again after a day or two. If the symptoms of paralysis are reduced or better, you may have found the trigger. If not, add the thing you removed or reduced back into the meal, etc. Then repeat and change something else:
- ❖ Change only one thing at that time:
  - ➢ Remove sugar or
  - ➢ Cut medication dose or
  - ➢ Stop or reduce the activity
    - ▪ Less than usual
    - ▪ Shorter than usual
- ❖ Repeat until you find the trigger or triggers.

Some suggestions for how to avoid the triggers once they are found:

- ➢ On feet too long? : Break the activity in several shorter periods on feet.
- ➢ Cannot eat sugar? : Stop and try sweeteners, honey, stevia, etc.
- ➢ Cannot eat certain food? : Find replacement or do without.
- ➢ Cannot take medication? : Cut dosage, stop taking or get a replacement (under supervision of medical professional).
- ➢ Sitting too long? : Get up every hour or less and move around.
- ➢ Sitting too long? : Exercise in chair.
- ➢ Dehydrated? : Drink more water, set timer.
- ➢ Hungry? : Eat several smaller meals.
- ➢ Too hot? : Wear looser, cooler clothes, use neck cooler.
- ➢ Too cold? : Add clothing layers, use a blanket, drink hot drinks.
- ➢ Cannot drink caffeine: Drink decaffeinated drinks.

As the triggers are discovered and eliminated the attacks of paralysis and other associated symptoms will begin to decline. The quality of life will improve. The information will be recorded and can be shared with the doctors and used as a tool during the diagnosing process. Use the following blank page to record your own triggers as you discover them.

My Known Triggers

Identify And Eliminate Triggers

Monitoring the Triggers and Symptoms

Once many of the triggers have been established and a diagnosis has been obtained (or not), it will be necessary to continue to observe and monitor the symptoms and the triggers. As we have discovered from my our experience and that of others with Periodic Paralysis, the triggers may change over time or what may have seemed to be the cause, may not actually be the cause. It is important to keep track continually in order to regulate and control the symptoms.

For instance, at first it may appear that sugar eaten in a cookie is the culprit causing attacks of muscle weakness or paralysis. Later it may be discovered that it was actually the white flour or the chocolate in a cookie that may have caused the episode. Accidentally, it may be figured out that a person might be able to eat small amounts of sugar in a gluten-free cookie. Then after eating the gluten free cookie everyday for three days, a paralytic episode occurs. This may be that too much was eaten. So, it may be that small amounts of sugar may be eaten occasionally, just not everyday.

It is a fine line that an individual with Periodic Paralysis must walk everyday. We must move through life as if we are walking a tightrope. It has been said that when we figure out what our triggers are, we must treat them as if they are allergies, something we must avoid. However, it becomes a problem when those things are important elements needed in the body such as salt or sugar.

In discussion with other individuals, we also have discovered that surprising things may actually cause an attack. We may believe we are doing everything correctly and avoiding all triggers and then we suddenly slip into full body paralysis. This happened to me recently. I tripped on my oxygen cord and landed on my knees. I scraped up one of them, but otherwise felt fine. Three hours later I was in full body paralysis.

After discussing this with a friend and wondering what had caused this attack, he reminded me that adrenaline is released when the body is stressed or experiences some trauma. I realized that although I did not notice much when I fell except a small scrape to my knee, my body had recognized it as trauma, released adrenaline and three hours later I was paralyzed and for the following several days.

Now I will remember that if I fall again, no matter how small or uneventful it may seem, I must prepare for the possibility of slipping into paralysis. I will be sure to rest and hope it will neither happen again nor be as serious as the last time. Better yet, I need to be more careful, now that I know if I fall, I will go into paralysis (or break a bone knowing I have severe osteoporosis).

Monitoring or keeping track of triggers is important because it seems as if they are always changing and maybe they are or maybe it is the amount of something we are using, but also it may be that we have misinterpreted one trigger for another. We must use the charts to keep track of symptoms and possible triggers and put them together in a journal. The information in the charts and journal will be recorded and can be shared with the doctors and used as a tool during the diagnosing process or for treatment options.

Eleven
Relieve Your Symptoms
CHANGING LIVES NATURALLY

- ❖ **Relieve your symptoms**
  - ➢ **Avoid all known triggers**
    - **Medications**
    - **Stress**
  - ➢ **Eat a pH balanced diet**
  - ➢ **Avoid processed foods**
  - ➢ **Use organic foods**
  - ➢ **Drink distilled water**
  - ➢ **Use organic natural supplements**
  - ➢ **Stay well rested**
  - ➢ **Stay well hydrated**
  - ➢ **Avoid physical exercise and exertion**
  - ➢ **Avoid heat and cold**
  - ➢ **Treat Paralysis**
    - **Take potassium or not**
    - **Take glucose or carbohydrates or not**
    - **Use oxygen during paralysis**
    - **Do nothing**
  - ➢ **Use meditation and mental imagery**

Introduction

As discussed in previous chapters of this book, we know that individuals with Periodic Paralysis, suffer greatly from many symptoms such as partial or total paralysis, heart arrhythmias or muscle weakness brought on by any number of triggers such a sugar, stress or carbohydrates. This chapter contains the most important components for the relief, treatment or management of those symptoms. Due to the fact that I am unable to take any type of medication, this plan is based on and uses mostly natural methods and substances in order to reduce the attacks of paralysis and other symptoms.

Calvin and I created our plan after a great deal of research and much trial and error over a period of several years.

Avoid All Known Triggers

The most obvious and common sense step that can easily be done to relieve our symptoms is to avoid the triggers known to cause them. Some are very obvious and others may take some time to discover. (Sometimes you may never know what sets an attack into motion.) Chapter Ten discusses the most obvious and common triggers and how to discover the triggers that set off a paralytic attack or other symptoms. Referring to those chapters will be helpful to know what to avoid. The following is more in depth discussion of some of the more common triggers and why they create symptoms and paralysis in Periodic Paralysis.

Medications/Over-the-Counter Medications

It is best to remember that most medications including over-the-counter are triggers. If you are taking prescribed medications, it is important to discuss this issue with the doctor. Do not attempt to stop taking prescribed medications without the care of a physician. Many pharmaceuticals may produce very serious complications if stopped suddenly. Tapering off slowly is the best method, however, even slowly withdrawing from a medication may cause unexpected symptoms. If a person needs to begin a new medication it is best to begin with one quarter of the amount prescribed until it is known if the body will tolerate it. Sometimes there is a delayed reaction and it may take a few weeks before symptoms occur.

Before I was diagnosed, the drugs that were given to me for all of the wrong diagnoses, created new symptoms, which caused more prescriptions until I was taking 15 different drugs. I had a huge seizure-like episode and nearly died. I had to be totally cared for because I could do nothing for myself and I had to regain enough strength to walk again. I have never fully recovered. If something were to happen to Calvin, I would have to live in an assisted living program. Then long QT interval heartbeats from taking two different antibiotics nearly killed me again. When I finally got my diagnosis and was prescribed the usual drugs given for PP, I nearly died a third time. Those of us with Periodic Paralysis must be very careful with all drugs of any kind, IV's, anesthesia and over the counter meds. Periodic Paralysis is a mineral metabolic disorder and therefore we do not react normally to drugs.

The two most common issues with drugs or pharmaceuticals for individuals with Periodic Paralysis are a paradoxical reaction and an idiosyncratic reaction. These are both serious effects. If one has a paradoxical reaction to a medication it means that the opposite of what is supposed to happen will occur. For instance, if someone takes a sleeping pill and then stays awake all night, it is known as a paradoxical effect. This can be just an inconvenience or very serious depending on the medical issue and the reaction. If someone who is already experiencing high blood pressure, is prescribed a drug to lower blood pressure, but it increases the blood pressure, this can cause a stroke, other serious effects or even death.

If an individual develops tremors, metabolic acidosis and paralysis from taking an antibiotic; these would be considered as idiosyncratic effects; reactions or side effects, which would be totally unpredicted, unexpected and never seen before. These effects would not be listed as possible rare side effects. This is a serious problem because these idiosyncratic effects, also known as "type B reaction" can be harmful by causing damage or even death. The amount ingested has no bearing on it. The reactions may occur from the smallest amount possible after one dose and the reactions may occur right away or after a little passage of time, even after a few weeks or chronically after a period of time

We want you to be safe and the best you can be, naturally!!!

The following are links to articles I wrote related to drugs and Periodic Paralysis:

http://livingwithperiodicparalysis.blogspot.com/2013/12/idiosyncratic-and-paradoxical-reactions.html
http://livingwithperiodicparalysis.blogspot.com/2013/12/why-people-with-some-forms-of-periodic.html
http://livingwithperiodicparalysis.blogspot.com/2013/11/pharmaceuticals-are-not-answer-for-some.html
http://livingwithperiodicparalysis.blogspot.com/2014/02/periodic-paralysis-and-anesthesia.html
http://livingwithperiodicparalysis.blogspot.com/2014/02/some-forms-of-pp-worsened-by-diamox.html
http://livingwithperiodicparalysis.blogspot.com/2014/06/beware-of-off-label-drugs.html

The Periodic Paralysis Guide And Workbook

Stress

Discover The Sources Of Stress And Seek Options To Deal With Them

Avoiding stress of all types is extremely important. This is difficult because it includes "good" stress such as celebrating holidays and attending or planning birthday parties. Strong emotions such as excitement, fear, panic and anger should be avoided because they cause the body to produce adrenaline, also known as epinephrine, and release it into the bloodstream. For some individuals with Periodic Paralysis the release of epinephrine triggers paralytic episodes because it lowers the amount of potassium in the blood. Illness or injury in the body also causes stress. Temperature extremes (heat and cold) and fasting or going without eating all put stress on the body and need to be avoided by some individuals. Adrenaline also produces an increase in the heart rate; blood pressure, blood sugars and irregular heart beats as well as paralysis.

Besides avoiding stress, learning how to deal with stress can also be helpful in bypassing symptoms and paralysis in the event of anxiety, fear, distress or tension. There are many ways of avoiding stress and handling it in a more acceptable and tolerable manner. We have created a plan to aid in avoiding these things and developing better coping skills.

The plan for dealing with stress must first begin with discovering its triggers in our daily lives. We can do this by creating a stress journal and writing in it everyday or as the events present themselves. We need to answer the following questions. What causes your stress? How did it make you feel? How did you respond? How did you make yourself feel better? How can you avoid the stressor? What options are available for the future?

Writing in a journal and answering these questions can help us to reduce and prevent our stress and to learn to cope better with our daily anxieties and tensions, thus minimizing or avoiding our symptoms and paralysis. We have created a form to be used as a guide in a daily journal. This form can also be copied and used in a loose-leaf folder. The plan follows.

Stress Management Plan

- Create a stress journal:
    - Write in it daily or as needed.
        - What caused your stress?
        - How did it make you feel?
        - How did you respond?
        - How did you make yourself feel better?
        - What options are available for the future?
            - Avoid or Change
                - Avoid stressful situations or triggers
                - Change the situation
                    - Learn to say "no"
                    - Back away from conflict
                    - Learn to "ask for help"
            - Adjust or Accept
                - Find different, new or better ways to do things
                - Seek therapy to cope with what cannot be changed
                - Join support groups
                - Utilize Natural Stress Reducers

Relieve Your Symptoms

Stress Journal

Cause Of Stress:

_____
_____
_____
_____

How Did It Make You Feel?

_____
_____
_____
_____

How Did You Respond?

_____
_____
_____
_____

How Did You Make Yourself Feel Better?

_____
_____
_____
_____

How To Avoid This Stressor?

_____
_____
_____
_____

Options or Alternatives?

_____
_____
_____
_____

Stress Reducers?

_____
_____
_____
_____

Periodic Paralysis Network, Inc. Sequim, Washington U.S.A. All rights reserved. Copyright © 2014

When filling out the Stress Journal Form first identify your personal stressors. Are there certain people, places, or situations that cause stress for you? How do these people, places or situations make you feel? Do you feel fear, anger, or anxiety? How do you respond to these feelings? Do you cry, argue or get depressed? Does it cause your physical symptoms and paralysis? How do you make yourself feel better? Do you overeat, smoke or ignore the situation? How do you avoid the stressor? Can you avoid the stressor? What are your other options or alternatives to these things? Can you avoid the people, stay away from the places or situations that create the stress? Can you change them? If it is not possible to avoid or change the situation, can you change how you feel about them? Can you adapt or adjust to the situation? Can you adapt or adjust by using stress-reducing methods? Once you identify your stressors in your journal and understand how they affect you, it is time to decide what to do about them. You can avoid, change, adjust or accept them. You can also use stress reducers and relaxation to cope better with those things that cannot be changed.

Change or Avoid: Avoid the stressors - If not, **change** them.
　Make new friends
　Get a new doctor
　Change your diet

Adjust or Accept: Accept people, things and situations as they are - If not, **adjust**.
　Find new, different or better ways to do things.
　Attend therapy or counseling to learn to cope, accept or adjust.
　Join support groups. Get support and understand better things you cannot change.

Cope Using Stress Reducers And Relaxation Ideas

Natural Stress Reducers And Coping Skills:
- Get enough sleep
- Eat right
- Get up periodically
- Write thoughts in journal
- Talk it out
- Arrange for private time
- Plan ahead
- Do not procrastinate
- Write everything down
- Ask questions
- Relax standards
- Count your blessings
- Turn off phone
- Talk yourself through it
- Laugh it off
- Get organized
- Do something you enjoy
- Live one day at a time
- Become more flexible
- Be willing to compromise
- Be optimistic
- Develop patience
- Learn to say "no"
- Learn to say "yes"
- Learn to ask for help
- Back away from conflict
- Allow extra time

Relaxation Strategies:
- Music
- Meditate
- Call a friend
- Take a nap
- Go for a walk
- Read a book
- Light yoga
- Deep breathing
- Aromatherapy
- Exercise if possible
- Use guided imagery
- Get a massage
- Spend time with a pet
- Create an art project
- Play a game
- Drink a healthy tea
- Cuddle with someone
- Go outside
- Enjoy a hobby
- View a good movie
- Watch television
- Take a bath
- Do a puzzle
- Draw or paint

Diet and Nutrition
Make Healthy Lifestyle Changes

Lifestyle changes are difficult at first, but the results are well worth the effort. I have regained my life in most ways by avoiding the triggers of my paralytic episodes and by changing how and what I eat.

Many of us with various forms of Periodic Paralysis cannot get medications and/or cannot take them. A few years ago I was basically dying due to this fact. Calvin and I researched and experimented and discovered the best way to reduce my periods of full body, total paralysis lasting hours at a time and occurring four to five times a day and all night, was with a pH balanced diet, also know as an alkaline diet. We added supplements and I avoided all of my triggers except sleep (have to sleep) and began to use oxygen for my exercise intolerance.

By the end of 6 months, my episodes were reduced to one or two a month and I had lost 25 pounds, my A1C levels were down to normal ranges and my cholesterol levels had been reduced significantly. I was able to function more normally and continue to be much better than when I started the diet three years ago. Now that I have become balanced, I find I have needed to add a bit more salt, sugar, carbohydrates and fats and am able to cut back on the supplements.

We have adopted several sayings when it comes to eating:

- *"Eat to live rather than live to eat."*
- *"Eat from the farm and not the factory."*
- *"Eat 70 percent alkaline and 30 percent acidic."*

The 70/30 eating rule is the most important of the group. We have it posted on our refrigerator along with the acid and alkaline ratings of particular foods.

Periodic Paralysis is not curable but we believe it is manageable, in part, by the things we consume and the things we avoid. Highly acidic chemicals and food can trigger potassium shifting. The relationship between potassium shifting and metabolic acidosis is quite real and should be taken very seriously in order to avoid life-threatening complications. The goal is consume much more alkaline and much less acid.

Eat a Proper pH Balanced Diet
"Eat to live rather than live to eat"

When Calvin discovered I had metabolic acidosis and was unable to take any medication, he began to search for ways to save my life. He had discovered that the pH balance in my body was unbalanced with too much acidity. He set out to increase the alkaline in my body. He found a website with a chart containing the pH balance of the most common foods. With the chart in hand, he hurried to the store and bought as many of the foods containing alkaline he could find, mostly vegetables. Then he found our juicer and made a vegetable and fruit drink for me every morning, he prepared fresh vegetables for my lunch and made a fresh salad for my dinner. He cut out almost all foods with acidity. It was difficult for me so he decided to eat the same diet with me. Soon I was doing better. I grew stronger, the attacks of paralysis decreased in number and severity and by the time six months had passed, we both lost twenty pounds and our cholesterol levels were decreased and sugar levels were down in the normal ranges.

While attending a visit with one of my diagnosing doctors, we told him about the diet and how it had helped me. He said that we were now, "Eating to live and no longer living to eat." He was so right!

What we had discovered was the body has a natural pH balance. It is 70% alkaline and 30% acidic. Any deviation from this may cause an imbalance. Any imbalance in the body causes stress and may trigger symptoms or paralysis. If the body becomes too acidic, metabolic acidosis may occur. Too much alkaline in the body can also be a serious problem causing dehydration. With this in mind, each meal eaten should contain 70% alkaline food and 30% acidic food. There are several good websites on the Internet with charts listing foods high in acidity and high in alkaline. These sites also have instructions for how to follow the diet and recipes for preparing healthy dishes. Links to these sites can be found on our website Periodic Paralysis Network.

Unprocessed Foods
"Eat from the farm; not the factory"

The best way to follow a pH balanced diet is to remember to, "Eat from the farm; not from the factory." This is because most junk food and processed foods are packed with substances, which are acidic or naturally more acidic. Meat is also a more acidic food. Another way to remember how to shop in order to keep the body pH balance is to stay out of the center isles in the grocery store. The good and healthy foods are always on the outer lanes of the store.

That being said, it is best to remember the word "balance." It is easy to be afraid to eat too much alkaline and forget to eat the 30% acidity. With that in mind, and remembering an individual's triggers, some food with acidity is permitted.

Organic Foods

We suggest that when purchasing the food for the pH balanced diet it should be organically grown and processed as much as possible. There are several reasons. The most important is to avoid additives, hormones and pesticides, which can possibly be triggers. If not triggers, they may cause illness and indirectly be triggers for paralytic attacks.

Most cows and cattle (and other animals we eat) are given hormones and antibiotics, unless organically raised. The dairy products and meat from these animals will contain a certain amount of them. If antibiotics or hormones are triggers for an individual, he or she may not be aware that those will be found in the milk, cheese or meat they eat. Without realizing it they may be ingesting them, thus creating episodes of paralysis and not knowing why.

Distilled Water

The same thing applies to our drinking water. The hormones, antibiotics and other medications passed from humans and animals into our water supply are remaining even

after the water is purified. Individuals with Periodic Paralysis may not realize they are actually ingesting these medications, hormones and antibiotics in drinking water. For this reason, we suggest using a distiller to process drinking water. It is the only way to have pure drinking water, unless the water is from a good well, which has been tested and found free of all contaminants.

Nutrient Extractor

Extracting nutrients from natural food sources is much more affordable and convenient today with the use of a nutrients extractor. NutriBullet is the kitchen tool we use to turn raw vegetables, fruits, nuts and seeds into liquid drinks that help optimize metabolism, overall health and pH balance on the alkaline side.

Balance

"Balance" is the most important word in our plan. If just one thing is out of balance, it can mean the difference between life and death in some cases. Besides the 70/30 balances in our diet, the other elements in our body must be in balance also, especially the elements or minerals (sometimes called electrolytes). This is due to the fact that Periodic Paralysis is a mineral metabolic disorder and when the minerals are out of balance, paralysis will occur. Some of these elements are calcium, magnesium, sodium, potassium, chloride, and bicarbonate.

That being said, however, salt (sodium) may be a trigger for paralytic episodes for most individuals. Due to that fact many of us avoid it like the plague. If we do not eat any salt then our body will get out of balance and episodes of paralysis or other symptoms may develop. So we must carefully ingest some sodium for that balance.

This also includes natural sugar and some fats and oils. These are also needed in our body, but care must be given to how much we eat of them in our diet and which types. Natural sugars in fruits would be a better choice than white processed table sugar. Olive oil is a better choice than vegetable oil. Monounsaturated fats and polyunsaturated fats are a better choice than saturated fats.

I discovered these things the hard way. After many months of not eating salt, sugar, carbohydrates and fats and oils, and experiencing great improvement with almost no paralytic episodes, I suddenly got very ill and began to have more episodes of severe paralysis. I became extremely weak and overall quite ill. After researching it, I discovered I was probably suffering from too much alkalinity and an imbalance of electrolytes and my body needed some sugar and some fats. I decided that I needed to carefully re-introduce these things back into my diet, one at a time to monitor for problems. I began to feel better, the paralytic episodes decreased and I regained my strength. I am still very careful, but I now enjoy better balanced diet. "Balance" is the key!

The pH Balanced Diet
"Eat 70 percent alkaline and 30 percent acidic."

We are often asked to describe the pH balanced diet discussed in our book *living with Periodic Paralysis: The Mystery Unraveled*, also known as the alkaline diet. Before discussing this diet we must first explain that there are different diets typically recommended for Hypokalemic Periodic Paralysis and Hyperkalemic Periodic Paralysis. The diet recommended for Hypokalemic Periodic Paralysis is basically a low sodium, low carbohydrate and high potassium diet. The recommended diet for Hyperkalemic Periodic Paralysis is basically a high carbohydrate, low potassium and low sodium diet. For all types of PP fasting should be avoided and care should be taken to avoid dips or increases in sugar levels. It is important to remember, however, that Periodic Paralysis is a mineral metabolic disorder and our bodies can easily become out of balance. So keeping the above diet guidelines in mind, we must also keep our pH levels in balance.

The most important thing to remember is the 70%-30% part of the diet. This means 70% alkaline and 30% acid. Then you must factor in the organic and natural issues. There are many websites that have charts, recipes and menus for the alkaline diet also known as the pH diet. The 70/30 is the balance between acidity and alkaline that our body must maintain to keep us alive and well. If we are too acidic or too alkaline we become ill as discussed earlier.

The foods with the most alkaline are fresh green vegetables, grasses, sprouts, peas, beans, lentils, spices, herbs and seasonings, and seeds and nuts (mainly almonds). Foods that are more acidic (eat sparingly) are meat, fish, poultry, dairy products, eggs, grains, and legumes.

Balance is the important word when it comes to putting a meal together and for snacking. We also need to remember the sugar, salt (sea) and oil/fat content of the foods we eat. Do not entirely eliminate them just use sparingly. Processed foods have these things and chemicals so eat as fresh and organic as possible.

I cannot eat gluten and try to use dairy products sparingly, so my diet is even more restricted. I eat a great deal of raw vegetables and salads.

A salad will contain greens, tomatoes, avocados (at each meal if possible) cucumbers, carrots, celery, sprouts, mushrooms, peppers, nuts (almonds), seeds (pumpkin and sunflower) all about 70% and then I add a few things like, a few bites of chicken or beef or pork, maybe some cheese, a few olives and olive oil and vinegar or lemon (30%).

I use a NutriBullet and add a mixture of 30/70 including nuts and seeds and coconut milk.

In my refrigerator I have a mixture of shredded fresh beets (purple and/or golden), carrots, turnips, rutabagas and parsnips. When I want a snack or even for breakfast, I put some in a bowl and add some oil and vinegar and eat it just like that or sometimes I add some nuts, raisins and dried coconut with some low fat sour cream (organic). I also put some on my salads.

Relieve Your Symptoms

I buy many vegetables and have them washed and cut and in containers ready to grab when I need or want a snack.

For my dinners, I usually eat a big salad, or a 70/30 meal. 70% vegetables (which can be cooked but best if raw due to becoming more acidic when cooked or processed) that can be a small salad, sometimes some sweet potato or regular potato (with butter; it is neutral pH) a few bites of meat/fish/poultry. I do occasionally make a casserole type meal keeping in mind the 70/30 rules. Stir-fry dishes are easy to make into a 70/30.

My biggest problem is trying to do breakfast at 70/30. Oatmeal or brown rice is not the best but I add nuts, seeds, coconut and dried fruit or fresh berries. A nice salad for breakfast is another option.

Occasionally I add some of my favorite acidic things in a (or to a) meal as part of the 30%. This way I do not feel deprived. I can eat some things I enjoy and I am not missing out on what everyone else or Calvin is eating.

I will use pasta (brown rice or corn or a mixture of both) to make spaghetti and then eat more of the sauce and vegetables or a salad. In that way I do not feel cheated or left out.

You can basically eat whatever you want that is not a trigger as long as you use the 70/30 rules. It is just incorporated into the 30% part of the meal.

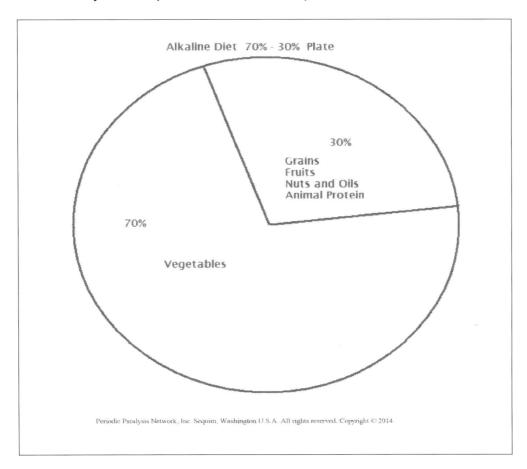

The chart illustrates how the proportions of food should look on the plate.

Many wonderful and delicious recipes can be found on the Internet under "alkaline diet recipes" or "pH balance diet recipes."

The following are links to articles related to diet and Periodic Paralysis:

http://livingwithperiodicparalysis.blogspot.com/2014/04/standard-healthy-eating-is-not-best-for.html

http://livingwithperiodicparalysis.blogspot.com/2013/11/periodic-paralysis-diet-november-25-2013.html

The weekly diet chart should be an aide with meal planning. The alkaline diet takes some time for planning, purchasing and preparing the food. It is best to have it all done ahead of time and ready to easily grab as needed. Be sure to allow yourself enough time for these things in order to avoid or reduce stress.

Besides shopping in specialty stores and cooking from scratch, you may also decide use things like a sprouter for seeds and beans, or a food dehydrator. You can even choose to grow your own organic garden!

Notes_____
_____
_____
_____
_____
_____
_____
_____
_____
_____
_____
_____
_____
_____
_____
_____
_____
_____
_____
_____
_____
_____
_____
_____
_____
_____

Alkaline Diet 70% - 30% Weekly Planning Chart
Periodic Paralysis Network, Inc. Sequim, Washington U.S.A. All rights reserved Copyright © 2014

	Monday	Tuesday	Wednesday	Thursday	Friday	Saturday	Sunday
Breakfast							
Lunch							
Dinner							
Snacks							
Drinks							

Supplements

No matter how many vegetables, nuts, and sprouts we consume, we may not ingest all of the vitamins and minerals our bodies need to function optimally on a daily basis. This leaves us with the question of whether or not to take supplements? The whole idea of taking dietary supplements runs contrary to everything we have said about eating natural substances originating directly from the farm and avoiding processed foods made in a factory. Dietary supplements are a product of some form of factory processing, but there are exceptions to the rules.

Taking dietary supplements might just be the exception to the rule because the potential benefits outweigh the deficits depending on the supplement. Supplements come in all shapes, sizes, forms, and containers each with multitudes of claims. How do we separate out fact from fiction? Research is the only way to identify honest from dishonest claims. Many people take supplements in the form of a pill and other people use liquids and powders.

I chose to take supplements in powder form along with a glass of fresh vegetable and fruit juice made with our juicer or NutriBullet. This works for us but might not work for everyone else. It is a personal choice. We read labels and verify claims using the Internet. We avoid preservatives and unnecessary additives. We avoid capsules and hard-shelled pills. We avoid non-organic vitamin and mineral sources. Research helps us make informed and healthy choices. It all takes time and a commitment to living a healthier lifestyle.

We have discovered several trusted Internet based businesses with quality supplements that can be bought in bulk such as potassium bicarbonate, potassium citrate, calcium citrate, and magnesium citrate. Since I am unable to take any antibiotics because it causes paralysis, I use herbs to treat bacterial infections and takes probiotics to help avoid infections. We are learning to use natural herbs to help boost our natural immune system. The businesses with quality supplements and herbs we trust can be found on our website Periodic Paralysis Network.

Stay Well-Rested

It is extremely important for individuals with Periodic Paralysis to stay well rested. Otherwise an individual's body becomes stressed and stress equals paralysis. A full night of sleep is essential. Unfortunately, many are affected by paralysis at night because different phases of sleep are a trigger. Falling asleep, during sleep and waking up may trigger a paralytic episode. It is best to do everything possible to make those times, stress free, comfortable and temperature controlled to make it less likely to trigger an episode.

There are many methods that may aid in falling asleep, getting better sleep and staying asleep. Using the following strategies may be helpful. The following issues are covered; comfort of the bedroom in every way, things to do and not do before going to bed, what to do and not do at bedtime and what to do once you get in bed and cannot fall asleep. It is best to experiment to discover what will work.

Relieve Your Symptoms

Strategies For Naturally Falling Asleep More Quickly:

- ❖ **Bedroom Comfort:**
    - ➢ Comfortable bed
        - Too hard
        - Too soft
        Comfortable bedding
        - Too many blankets
        - Not enough blankets
        - Sheets flannel
        - Sheets light and airy
        - Sheets dense and silky
    - ➢ Comfortable temperature
        - Cooler room 60 to 67 degrees
        - Warmer room
        - Window open
        - Window shut
        Comfortable position
        - On side
        - Pillow between legs
    - ➢ Comfortable bedclothes
        - Flannel
        - Light and airy
        - Dense and silky flannel
    - ➢ Light
        - Eliminate all light
            - Night-lights
            - Clocks
            - Electronics
            - LED
            - Mask
    - ➢ Sound
        - Eliminate all possible noises
            - Use earplugs
    - ➢ Aromatherapy
        - Lavender

- ❖ **Before Bedtime:**
    - ➢ Warm bath
    - ➢ Journal two hours before bed or
    - ➢ Write a worry list
        - Prevents mind racing later
    - ➢ Relaxation techniques
    - ➢ Warm drink
        - Milk
        - Herbal tea
    - ➢ Read
    - ➢ Word games or puzzles

- Television
- Be well hydrated
- Be well fed

❖ **At Bedtime:**
- Routine
  - Same time to sleep, same time to rise
- Cannot sleep?
  - Get up and do something
  - Read
  - Word games or puzzles
  - Television

❖ **In Bed:**
- Adjust pillows
- Meditate
- Imagery
- Visualize a "happy place"
  - Beach
  - Forest
  - Lake
- Progressive relaxation
  - Start with head
  - Move to toes
- Squeeze and relax muscles
- Deep breathing techniques
- Curl and uncurl toes
- Calming music
  - Ambient sounds
    - Running water
    - Rain
    - White noise
- Count blessings
- Count backwards
- Replay entire day in head

Notes_____
_____
_____
_____
_____
_____
_____
_____
_____
_____

Relieve Your Symptoms

Stay Well Hydrated
Drink Plenty of Water

Being chronically ill leaves individuals more susceptible to dehydration, which is when the body loses more liquid than it takes in. Less water and fluids affects the balance of the electrolytes and prevents the organs from working properly. This creates an imbalance, which creates stress in the body. As we know, stress can trigger paralysis.

The most important way to stay hydrated is to drink plenty of water and other healthy liquids.

Physical Exercise and Exertion
Exercise Intolerance and Permanent Muscle weakness

Most individuals with all forms of Periodic Paralysis usually avoid physical exercise, physical exertion, weight lifting, heavy labor and physical therapy. This is due to exercise intolerance and/or gradual permanent muscle weakness (PMW).

The recurring episodes of paralysis cause damage to the muscles, thus creating exercise intolerance leading to gradual muscle weakness and over time Permanent Muscle Weakness (PMW) results. The damage done to the muscles is written about much less often than the episodes of partial or full paralysis in articles or studies about Periodic Paralysis. The information available, however, indicates that PMW is seen in all forms of PP, Hypokalemic Periodic Paralysis, Hyperkalemic Periodic Paralysis, Normokalemic Periodic Paralysis or Andersen-Tawil Syndrome. Progressive muscle damage is also seen in all forms and it is irreparable. It cannot be reversed. This overlooked subject is extremely important and needs to be addressed. Each paralytic episode causes more muscle damage so it is necessary to do everything possible to stop the episodes.

There are two types of involvement of muscles in individuals with Periodic Paralysis. There are attacks of paralysis of the muscles, which are intermittent, and there is a myopathy or a progressive, permanent muscle weakness, which can occur. Some individuals experience one or the other and some experience both conditions, though it is less common to have both, and it is very rare to have only the progressive, permanent muscle weakness. If an individual develops the progressive, permanent form of periodic paralysis, it begins as exercise intolerance, usually in the legs and feet, which progressively spreads to the rest of the muscles in the body.

In exercise intolerance the individual is not able to do physical exercise or exertion that would be expected from someone of his or her age and overall health level nor for the amount of time expected. He or she lacks stamina. The individual may also experience extreme pain and fatigue after exercising or exertion and other symptoms such as a feeling of heaviness in the muscle groups. Exercise intolerance is a symptom rather than a condition or disease. It is a common symptom found in several diseases including metabolic disorders. Periodic Paralysis is a mineral metabolic myopathy.

Food and oxygen are normally converted into energy and delivered to the muscles but this cycle is disrupted in individuals with exercise intolerance. The muscles are unable to use the nutrients and oxygen and therefore, enough energy may not be generated to the muscles and he or she is left with little or no energy. The degrees of low energy can be mild or extreme and the symptoms may occur during exercise or exertion or they can occur later, even the next day.

Symptoms of exercise intolerance include: fatigue, muscle cramps, insufficient heart rate, depression, changes in blood pressure and cyanosis. Fatigue may show within minutes of beginning to exercise with shortness of breath or dizziness. This is a sign that sufficient oxygen is not being processed. For individuals with severe exercise intolerance this can happen after doing simple tasks such as eating, sitting up in a chair or writing. Muscle cramping and stiffness also will appear within a few minutes of beginning to exercise. This can linger for days after the exercising. There may also be a delayed reaction of hours and the pain may begin while one is sleeping causing one to awaken. The heart rate does not increase enough to meet the needs of the muscles during the activity. Depression is often seen in individuals with exercise intolerance. Not being able to do the things a person wants to do or should be able to do can create anxiety, irritability, bewilderment and hopelessness leading to depression. Standing up or walking across a room may be all that is necessary for an individual's blood pressure to rise significantly. Cyanosis is a serious condition that indicates there is not enough oxygen in the blood. The individual may appear to look blue in the face and hands and needs immediate medical attention.

Exercise intolerance can be seen in the small muscle groups as well as the large muscle groups. Writing or other fine motor skills can be affected causing cramping, fatigue and spasms. Tachycardia (fast heart beats) can occur from increased breathing rate during exercise or exertion and this rapid breathing increase is from fatigue of the diaphragm and chest wall. Vision may become blurry due to fatigue of the eye muscles. The oral muscles, those involving the mouth, may be affected making speech difficult and making chewing of harder or tougher foods a problem.

During exercise, potassium levels increase. Then about three minutes after stopping, the potassium levels drop. This shifting is why exercise is a problem and a trigger for many with Periodic Paralysis. For those with Hyperkalemic Periodic Paralysis or Paramyotonia Congenita when the potassium shifts up it can set things into motion. If one has Hypokalemic Periodic Paralysis and the potassium drops it can set things into motion. For many with Normokalemic Periodic Paralysis, or those whose potassium shifts in normal ranges, this can also set off the symptoms. For many, the mere shifting of potassium alone, regardless of the direction, can set the symptoms or paralysis into motion. Those with Andersen-Tawil Syndrome have symptoms and paralysis from shifting both high and low and in normal ranges.

Another reason that exercise is a problem for those with PP is because it is stressful to the body and therefore, epinephrine, also known as adrenaline, is released into the bloodstream during exercise or exertion. Epinephrine is a trigger for paralysis.

Although exercise should be eliminated, warm water exercises, massage, acupuncture and other options may be helpful. Each person is different so seeking **knowledgeable** medical advice and trial and error to discover what will work is the best option.

Heat and Cold

Maintaining a balanced temperature in the environment is important for people with Periodic Paralysis. If an individual gets hot or chilled, the body becomes stressed and can trigger a paralytic episode. Being prepared for transitional times is the best idea. Some simple ideas for temperature fluctuations may include wearing several layers of clothing or having several layers easily available. Have blankets and throws easily available. Use an electric blanket to heat the bed and turn it off just before slipping in (especially for those who have a problem with EMF's). Or, use the clothes dryer to warm nightclothes and slip them on just before crawling into a cold bed or to warm clothes when dressing in the morning. Using a neck cooler when overheated or to prevent becoming overheated can really help. Keeping one ready in the refrigerator is helpful. (Instructions for making neck coolers can be found at the PPN website.) Either warming a car or cooling it before entering it can help avoid the drastic changes in temperature during the winter and summer months.

Treating Muscle Paralysis
"Potassium, Glucose or Nothing?"

For most individuals diagnosed with Periodic Paralysis or with symptoms of Periodic Paralysis, they know which type they have. It is either Hypokalemic Periodic Paralysis, which is low potassium levels, or Hyperkalemic Periodic Paralysis, which are high potassium levels or Normokalemic Periodic Paralysis in which potassium shifts mainly in normal ranges. Using a potassium reader (discussed in Chapter Five) can aid in discovering when the level of potassium in blood is too high or too low or within normal ranges). It is best to use the meter to know for sure what the levels are before medicating or taking potassium when symptoms begin. Chapter Four and Chapter Six contain lists of symptoms, which typically accompany different levels of potassium for those without a potassium reader.

Some individuals with low potassium levels use some off-label drugs for their respective symptoms and different types of potassium in different forms. Their paralysis is fairly well controlled. Others with high potassium issues also use the same off-label drugs to help alleviate their symptoms. They do not take potassium, because they already have too much and this would cause serious paralysis and metabolic acidosis. They can take glucose to help control the high amounts of potassium in their blood. Eating carbohydrates or trying to move around can also be helpful.

Individuals with Andersen-Tawil-Syndrome or Andersen-Tawil-Syndrome-"like" Periodic Paralysis must be extremely careful when taking potassium. Because, they have periods of high potassium and low potassium, it is essential to use a potassium reader to measure the amount in their blood when they begin to feel symptoms or use the list of symptoms to determine the level of potassium. Doing this, will assure that an individual will use the correct method by either taking potassium or eating some carbohydrates or by doing nothing.

Those with symptoms or paralysis while levels of potassium are in normal levels do not need to take potassium. It could cause a rise in potassium levels creating hyperkalemia.

Although most episodes of weakness and paralysis are frightening, especially in the beginning, most individuals will learn that once an episode begins, the best and only thing one can do is to stay calm and try to relax. However, it is best to have a caregiver monitor the vitals. If there is choking, heart arrhythmia, extreme blood pressure or heart rate or if breathing stops, then it may be necessary to call for paramedics. More information about when to call for an ambulance can be found in Chapter Fifteen.

Types of Potassium

When considering which type of potassium to use, it is important to understand the most common types; potassium bicarbonate, potassium citrate and potassium chloride. Potassium bicarbonate is a salty substance with no color or smell and it neutralizes acidity. Potassium citrate is also a salty substance. It is potassium bicarbonate, which has been combined with citric acid for faster absorption. It reduces acidity. Potassium chloride is also a salty substance created from a combination of potassium and chlorine. It will increase the acidity in the body.

It comes in many forms which include, salts, powders, liquid, and tablets. Some tablets may be released over time or some are easily dissolved. Liquid forms need to be diluted in water. The soluble tablets ad powder or salt forms need to be dissolved in water. Tablets should be swallowed whole with eight ounces of water after meals.

How does someone know which type and form is best for him or her? We are not medical doctors so we avoid offering advice about the type of potassium supplement to use. That needs to be discussed with your trusted medical advisor. However, that being said, the various forms and types are discussed here for a better understanding and decision-making.

After researching and knowing that I have chronic metabolic acidosis, I chose to use potassium bicarbonate because it neutralizes the acidity in my body. I use the salt form because and I can dilute it in water for quick absorption. I take it when my potassium levels are low. I must be careful with the amount I take because I easily swing into high potassium levels.

Although most individuals with Periodic Paralysis will get prescriptions for potassium, some may chose or need to purchase their own potassium supplements. If you purchase your own form be sure to use natural sources of potassium from a reliable natural organic source. The businesses with quality supplements which we trust for our needs can be found on our website Periodic Paralysis Network.

Use of Oxygen During Periods of Paralysis
"The Elephant on the Chest"

Oxygen should be handy to be used for anyone with Periodic Paralysis when in a paralytic episode because very often, an individual develops breathing issues. It can become difficult to breathe and it may feel like an elephant sitting on the chest. Breathing sometimes stops during an episode. Oxygen levels may drop and the person may develop hypoxia or inadequate oxygen levels. This can lead to respiratory arrest and death.

Oxygen should be used for individuals with Andersen-Tawil Syndrome or Andersen-Tawil Syndrome-like symptoms who are in paralytic episodes. An oximeter may not indicate the correct oxygen levels because of chronic or acute dilatation of the heart. This is an enlargement of the heart cavity. Death can occur.

Meditation and Mental Imagery
"I Am at Peace"

Paralytic attacks can be very frightening. They can last anywhere from a few minutes to several hours to days at a time. They can involve part of the body or the entire body. They may be severe or mild. Complications can arise such as breathing problems, heart arrhythmias, muscle cramping or choking. It may be difficult to remain calm during those times.

I know the fear involved and have spent many hours in full body paralysis, which involves not being able to see or speak or move in anyway. I experience choking, heart arrhythmias, chest pain, fluctuating heart rates (slow and fast) fluctuating blood pressure (high and low), difficulty breathing (slow and fast) and stoppage, severe muscle cramping, jerking, and pain, and fluctuating body temperatures with sweating and chills. All during this, I am still able to hear everything going on around me. On many occasions I was sure I was dying.

Over time, I have learned to relax to the best of my ability and just let it happen. I spend my time listening to the television or radio, whichever may be on, or the conversations going on among the people around me. I have also learned to meditate or use guided imagery.

When not in paralysis, I have taken time to learn how to meditate and enjoy guided imagery. I practice so it will come easy to me during an episode. I close my eyes and relax as I repeat, "I am" while I breathe in and "at peace" while I breathe out. I do this for several minutes.

Then I visualize being in my favorite place in the forest of pine and aspen trees, on a dirt path strolling beside a bubbling creek. I see squirrels and birds and an occasional deer. I see beautiful wildflowers of all colors along the path. The sky is always blue and the sun is always shining, the temperature is warm and I feel a slight breeze on my face. I continue to walk along the path and see new flowers, birds, trees and animals. I may meet someone on the trail. I may find things along the way.

Soon the episode has passed and I am able to open my eyes and I am able to begin moving once again. This has helped me to get through some very rough times. Anyone can adapt this to his or her own preferences, such as walking along the beach or enjoying a boat ride on a lake.

There are many websites on the Internet with scripts, audiotapes and videos of guided imagery that can be copied or downloaded for free. These also are available for learning how to meditate.

Conclusion

We believe this chapter to be one of the most important in our book because it contains our techniques based on research and trial and error for maintaining a "balance" in all aspects of life for individuals with Periodic Paralysis. With this method, some control may be regained in life by reducing the number and severity of the paralytic episodes and other symptoms and the debilitating complications experienced. We believe that by following the steps in this plan, which uses natural methods and common sense ideas, the cruel symptoms of Periodic Paralysis will be relieved for everyone who seriously attempts to stay balanced in order to 'walk the tightrope.' We believe you can 'be the best you can be naturally.'

Notes_____

Twelve
Find A Doctor
NOT EASY BUT POSSIBLE

- ❖ **Finding a Doctor**
  - ➢ Ask present doctors for names of doctors
  - ➢ Ask present doctors for referrals to doctors who may know about PP
  - ➢ Call insurance company
  - ➢ Call doctors' offices
  - ➢ Research on the Internet
  - ➢ Contact the nearest MDA
  - ➢ Think "outside the box"
  - ➢ Be creative

Finding a Doctor Who Cares

So many people with all forms of Periodic Paralysis struggle with locating doctors who can and will help them with both a diagnosis and proper treatment. They go from doctor to doctor and disappointment after disappointment, misdiagnosis after misdiagnosis and mistreatment after mistreatment. This can go on for decades with the misinformation following them from physician to specialist. Often, this will lead to a diagnosis of hypochondria, malingering or the archaic "conversion disorder" and a referral to a psychiatrist. Many of the patients become depressed and begin to doubt themselves after being prescribed medications for mental disorders that invariably make the symptoms worse or different, thus creating the need for yet another referral to yet another specialist.

As this vicious cycle continues over years, the symptoms worsen and the patient becomes more disabled and debilitated. Family and friends tire of dealing with the situation and many friends are lost, marriages end in divorce and family members withdraw their support. The patient is left in more pain and despair and the humiliation can be unbearable. Many are never diagnosed and never receive the treatment they need and deserve.

I myself saw thirty different medical professionals in six years before I was diagnosed at the age of 62 after a lifetime of illness, disability and loss of friends, family and a marriage. For the most part they were rude and did not understand what was happening to me. Most of them were frustrated and believed it to be all in my head. Five of these physicians were considered to be PP specialists.

Since finally getting diagnosed I have seen twelve more doctors, all of who do not know how to help me, including one who is a specialist in Andersen-Tawil Syndrome I also was able to finally locate a few doctors who have been willing to work with me (two more left town after seeing them for a short while) and have read the information I provided for them about Periodic Paralysis and done some research on their own. They do not deal directly with my PP symptoms, however, but with the things they know about, such as, diabetes, oxygen therapy and referrals to specialists as I need them.

After all of my experiences with finding doctors who will work with me, I have devised a common sense plan that can assist anyone to locate a doctor (Primary Care Physician: PCP) who will be willing to work with them before they ever step into the physician's office. There will be no more insults from a person who should be showing compassion and no more leaving the office in tears and despair.

1. The most obvious place to begin your search, if you have a good doctor who has decided to move on in his or her career, is to ask your present doctor for the name of a physician who knows about periodic paralysis or who would be willing to work with you. If he or she gives you a referral, be sure to have them confer with the new doctor about your disease and provide him with as much information as possible before your first visit. You may also want to provide information of your own ahead of time.

2. If you are not that lucky, the next thing you can do if you have insurance, is to call your insurance company and request a "patient advocate" or "case manager." Most insurance companies have employees whose job is to help their clients who have "more than the average" or "out of the ordinary" medical needs.

Once an advocate is assigned to you, you will need to explain your situation and Periodic Paralysis and explain your need to find a doctor who knows about the disease or who will be willing to work with you. It would be wise to seek out neurologists, internal medicine doctors and endocrinologists. You may need to see more than one doctor before you find the "right" one for you.

3. If your insurance company does not have patient advocates and has a restrictive list of particular doctors and specialists covered in their program, again, you will need to explain your situation and Periodic Paralysis and explain your need to find a doctor who knows about the disease or who will be willing to work with you. They will sometimes do the work for you.

If not, you can go through the lists of neurologists, endocrinologists or internal medicine doctors (experience indicates that regular medical doctors or family practitioners and even nurse practitioners actually are the most receptive) and call each office and ask for the office manager. You will need to explain your situation and Periodic Paralysis and explain your need to find a doctor who knows about the disease or who will be willing to work with you. In most cases, the office managers will speak to the doctor or doctors about your case and get back with you if the doctor is willing to see you.

4. If your insurance is not restrictive, you will have to check your local phone book or the web for neurologists, internal medicine doctors and endocrinologists in your area and proceed with the phone calling until you find one who will work with you.

Another good option, if your insurance is not restrictive and requires no referrals, is to check out the clinics in your area. The one I attend has 85 doctors and are connected to a local hospital. There should be at least one doctor willing to work with you.

You can proceed as explained previously; call and speak with one of the representatives. Explain your situation. The representative will go through the list of their recommended physicians and chose a few that may work for you. The doctors will be consulted and one or two may agree to see you. It may be wise to spend time with each to decide the "best fit" for you.

5. Without insurance, seeking out help from your local health department can be productive. Also your local services for disabled will have some possible options for finding a local doctor. You may be able to secure a social worker. He or she may do the work for or with you.

6. Thinking "outside of the box" can bring some surprises. I was so frustrated and about to give up on ever finding a local doctor who could diagnose and treat me, when I had a wild idea.

One of our local television stations offers a wonderful service every Tuesday evening during their two-hour news coverage. A local physician, and a guest specialist of her choosing, take calls from viewers and answer medical questions.

I called and asked if she knew about Periodic Paralysis. I was shocked when she told me she had a patient who had it and that the patient saw a local neurologist who treated her. She gave me the name of the neurologist. I made an appointment and after two visits was diagnosed! (I must explain that I had all of my medical records in hand with years of medical testing ruling everything else out and a referral from my nurse practitioner.)

7. The next option I offer must be used with caution. You may search the web for specialists. Seeking out these specialists in the field of Periodic Paralysis or Andersen-Tawil Syndrome, may lead you to some severe disappointment. There are several across the United States and a few around the world. Many do not see patients and are involved in research only.

The specialists will only diagnose based on genetics or a very "pure" form of the disease. (This may be based on the fact that most of them are researchers and their funding is based on working with only those who are genetically diagnosed. This leaves out a high percentage of us.) Their view can be extremely narrow and I have been surprised that their knowledge of the disease can be severely lacking in some areas. Their only option for treatment is limited to medications that do not work for many of us. If you have other conditions co-existing with your Periodic Paralysis or do not have a known genetic code, you will be sent packing in tears and humiliation. It is not worth the time or money you may spend to travel to another state or country.

Recently, I know of several individuals who had symptoms of Periodic Paralysis. They went to great expense to travel to the "specialists" only to be told that they absolutely did not have Periodic Paralysis. Within a few months, genetic testing proved that they did indeed have variants of Periodic Paralysis.

8. The Muscular Dystrophy Association (MDA) is an organization that treats patients with muscle diseases, and lists all the forms of periodic paralysis under that umbrella. In order to see their doctors you must already have a diagnosis or be referred for a diagnosis by a doctor. However, most of the doctors we have information about at the MDA Clinics do not know about Periodic Paralysis or Andersen-Tawil Syndrome. Most offices around the

country do not know about Periodic Paralysis. If you call for a referral or information, you will probably be told that they do not know what you are talking about. I have had to call many MDA offices around the country for patients to tell them that they do indeed treat Periodic Paralysis and Andersen-Tawil Syndrome patients. I refer them to this information at their own website.

Also, although you may already have a diagnosis, you must see their doctors and be re-diagnosed before you will receive any treatment or benefits offered. If the MDA doctor does not agree with your previous doctors due to their lack of knowledge of the disease or their narrow view based on old facts and research, you may lose your diagnosis. It is not worth the chance. That being said, there are some very good MDA doctors and some of our friends with Periodic Paralysis are having some success with the ones they are seeing.

In conclusion, many of the people with genetic mutations that have been located do have good doctors and receive good treatment for their particular forms of Periodic Paralysis. They are very lucky. Some of them can lead nearly normal lives.

I understand, however, it is difficult to find a doctor who will work with those of us who suffer from the effects of Periodic Paralysis, if we have not yet been diagnosed or those of us with variants for which no genetic mutation has been discovered yet, even if we have been diagnosed clinically (based on symptoms) or for those of us who have other diseases which co-exist with our form of PP. The truth is, very few of us will get any real help from a doctor even if we find one who knows about the disease and is kind, sympathetic and empathetic. This is due to the fact that most of us are unable to tolerate the known medications and the doctors do not know how to help us.

So, although I have a Primary Care Physician and several good specialists, Calvin and I are still left to deal with my episodes of paralysis and my other symptoms with no real help from the medical field. They do not know how to help me, but treat me well and look after the things they can; like my heart problems, power wheelchair, oxygen, diabetes strips, labs, etc. I appreciate and understand their lack of knowledge of such a rare and baffling disease. They trust us with the plan we have created after much research and trial and error.

Warning!

Avoid at all cost any doctor who seems at all skeptical about Periodic Paralysis. Once you see the "blank look" with glazed eyes, the "shoulder shrug," and the "I don't know about this." comment. Run; do not walk, as fast as possible, from this medical professional. Chances are the comments he puts in your records will follow you for a very long time and may taint other doctors' view of you. Once there is any kind of resistance, it is time to move on.

Remember that we "hire" doctors to work for us. We have the right to "fire" any doctor who is not working in our best interest or who is unsympathetic, uncaring, aloof, arrogant, egotistical, or abusive or who is misinformed about Periodic Paralysis. Doctors, who are in a hurry to diagnose with "conversion disorder" or a mental issue, are lazy and really need to admit that they just do not know what is wrong rather than to malign someone

Find A Doctor

who is severely ill and ruin their chance for seeking and receiving appropriate care. These doctors need to be reported for their inappropriate behavior and mistreatment.

Notes:_____

Finding a Doctor Checklist	Done
➢ Ask present doctors for names of doctors	
➢ Ask present doctors for referrals to doctors who may know about PP	

➢ Call insurance company:
  ▪ Tell your story
  ▪ Explain about PP
  ▪ Ask for a case manager or patient advocate to assist you	

➢ Call doctors' offices.
  ▪ Internal medicine
  ▪ Neurologists
  ▪ Endocrinologists
  ▪ Nephrologist
  ▪ Regular MD's
  ▪ Family Practitioners
  ▪ Nurse Practitioners
  ▪ Clinics in the area
  ▪ Local Health Department
     • Ask to speak to the office managers
     • Explain situation to them.
     • Explain PP to them
     • Ask them to refer the best doctor
     • Ask them to speak to doctors
     • Ask for a call back
     • Wait for their call back	

➢ Research on the Internet
  ▪ Ask on the PP message boards or support groups
  ▪ Check PP websites for lists of PP doctors
  ▪ Search for the university hospitals near you
  ▪ Search for specialists in channelopathies
  ▪ Search for specialists in PP
     • BUT: Be very careful
     • They may use narrow and out-dated data
     • They look for only "pure" cases for research
     • They may overturn a previous diagnosis	

➢ Contact the nearest MDA office to get a referral
  ▪ BUT: Be very careful
     • Many MDA clinics and doctors know nothing about PP
     • If they do, they do not always know enough to help
     • They may overturn a previous diagnosis	

➢ Think "outside the box"	
➢ Be creative	
More Ideas:	

Periodic Paralysis Network, Inc. Sequim, Washington U.S.A. All rights reserved. Copyright © 2014

Thirteen
Get A Diagnosis
HIT THEM WITH THE FACTS

- ❖ **Getting a Clinical Diagnosis**
  - ➢ The Plan
    - Process of elimination
      - Gather the facts
      - Lab work
      - Periods of paralysis, documented
      - EKGs
      - Oximeter recordings
      - Genetic testing?
      - Previous medical records
      - Chart the triggers
      - Document potassium use
      - Gather and chart family information

Introduction

There are two methods used for diagnosis of the various types of Periodic Paralysis; one is through a genetic test, which studies one's DNA. If a mutation is found the person receives a "genetic" diagnosis. If a person is diagnosed based on their symptoms, once all else has been ruled out, it is called a "clinical" diagnosis. Too many doctors will not give a clinical diagnosis once everything else has been ruled out and are eager to diagnose a person, especially women, with a mental disorder such as "conversion disorder" and then prescribe a psychotropic medication which makes the symptoms worse or can actually kill someone with certain forms of PP.

The truth about the genetic mutations for Periodic Paralysis and Andersen-Tawil Syndrome:

More than 40% of all individuals with Periodic Paralysis have a form, which has not yet been discovered and must therefore, be diagnosed clinically, based on symptoms and characteristics.

The other issue is that up to 50% of those with PP have potassium shifting in normal ranges, rather than low or high, which causes their symptoms. Without a test proving low or high potassium, some uniformed doctors refuse to diagnose although everything else is ruled out and there are clearly periods of muscle weakness and/or paralysis.

It is my belief that too much emphasis is placed upon the genetic testing, because only about one half us will have a genetic mutation if we are tested genetically. Diagnosis needs to be based on symptoms and characteristic once all else is ruled out.

Getting a clinical diagnosis, based on our symptoms, is the most important step we can take. Once it is on paper, we are at least believed for emergency care issues, hospitalizations, possible medications, school issues for children, insurance, validation, vindication, disability and much more.

It is an individual decision to do genetic testing once one has a clinical diagnosis and best made knowing all of the facts.

The Plan

Before I had a diagnosis and I was very ill, Calvin was beside himself with worry because of the severe paralytic episodes I was experiencing four and five times a day and every night. I was having difficulty breathing during them. He met with a technician for medical equipment when we were trying to get oxygen and he told her the story. She told him the best way to get the help we needed and a diagnosis was to, "Hit them (doctors) between the eyes with the facts." That is just what we did!! Based on that idea I have created the following plan for others to use to gain a diagnosis. I am presenting it in an outline format to make it easy to follow and to use as a checklist.

- ❖ You must **gather all of the facts**:
  - ➢ It is important for **everything else to be ruled out**. Your PCP and a neurologist do these, because most of the symptoms resemble neuromuscular disorders. The tests ruling everything else out might include but are not limited to:
    - Lab work of all types,
      - Blood
      - Urine
    - MRI's,
      - Brain
      - Spine
    - Spinal taps,
    - X-rays
    - EEGs
    - EMGs
    - EKGs
    - CMAPs
    - Muscle biopsy
      (Some of the tests above may show changes that can be markers for PP).
- ❖ Most doctors diagnosing PP want lab work showing either:
  - ➢ Paralysis during shifting in normal ranges
  - ➢ Paralysis during shifting in low potassium and/or,
  - ➢ Paralysis during shifting high potassium
    - This is done by obtaining serum potassium levels
      - May need to be done several times until a baseline is established

- Then during episodes every 5 to 10 minutes...not just one blood draw...there is no way to see the shifting otherwise.
- It may be necessary for hospitalization in order to do this while in the paralysis.
- May need to be done for more than 24 hours until each is documented, during the episodes.
- If the shifting is in the normal ranges, it may never show up during tests, unless it is done every few minutes.
  - 50% of PP patients may not have potassium shifting out of normal ranges
  - ATS patients may shift all three ways.
- However, the latest information for diagnosing PP based on potassium levels in blood serum is as follows:
  - The potassium in the blood does not always shift above or below normal ranges in 50% of patients experiencing muscle weakness or paralysis or it shifts so quickly that it cannot be measured. Doctors need to diagnose a patient with Periodic Paralysis based on the patient's symptoms, specifically, heart symptoms on an EKG and the muscle strength or weakness and history of episodes of paralysis.
- *** The information above needs to be shared with your doctors. Most do not understand these concepts. ***

❖ There needs to be periods of paralysis, either total or partial, which can be documented (or progressive, gradual, fixed muscle weakness, all other things ruled out).
  - Videotaping is the best way to do this.
  - It may be necessary for hospitalization in order for doctors to see an individual while in the paralysis.

Warning!
Under no circumstances should an individual provoke his or her symptoms or an episode of paralysis by omitting medication or ingesting foods or perform activities, which are known triggers. This is a very serious thing to do and can lead to death.

❖ ECGs or EKGs consistent with "ion channelopathy," Periodic Paralysis or Andersen Tawil Syndrome. For specifics see Heart Issues in Chapter Four.
  - Needs to be done while in the paralysis so it may need to be done for more than 24 hours until each is documented, during the episodes.
    - Holter Heart Monitors are the best method
❖ Oximeter (oxygen) recordings
  - Indicating, levels dropping during paralysis.
  - If in an advanced case of PP, it may show hypoventilation.

- ❖ Genetic testing is available
  - ➢ Not necessary, but helpful for treatment and prognosis
  - ➢ See Chapter One for Specifics for Genetic Diagnosing of all forms of PP
    - ▪ 40% to 50% of all people with PP do not have identified mutations. They have yet to be discovered.
- ❖ Gather all previous medical records.
  - ➢ Be sure to ask for all doctors' records from each appointment you attend.
  - ➢ Get all lab records, x-rays, hospitalizations, etc.
- ❖ Chart the triggers for the episodes.
  - ➢ See Chapter Ten
  - ➢ Documenting an increase of episodes after eating carbohydrates, after exercising or after taking certain medications is important for being able to control the episodes and letting the doctor see what the triggers are for a diagnosis.
- ❖ Documenting a reduction of episodes when using potassium is good. This can indicate the loss of potassium after shifting and may indicate low potassium levels.
- ❖ Gather as much medical information as possible from family members who may have symptoms similar to Periodic Paralysis. It has a hereditary component.
- ➢ If one suspects Andersen-Tawil Syndrome, gather as much medical information as possible from family members and note the characteristics/symptoms. Create a family flowchart with this information. Adding pictures can be helpful in demonstrating the characteristics. (See pages 189 & 190)
- ➢

Gather the Facts

The best way to gather all of the medical information needed for a diagnosis is to create a medical journal. This workbook can be used as your personal medical Periodic Paralysis journal by completing the forms and charts in Section Three and other forms throughout this book. It may stand alone or you can use it together with a three-ring loose-leaf folder and plenty of pocket files, designed to fit into the folder, to keep the loose testing results, doctor's office notes and other important forms. With good labeling in alphabetical order for each section, it can be organized to hold all of the medical records in an easy-to-locate manner. All of the charts and forms in this book have been designed to be scanned and can be used in another folder or notebook without this workbook, but I suggest you use them together.

The journal should contain your personal medical history and all testing results that indicate the probability of a form of Periodic Paralysis to include but not limited to lab reports, office notes (depending on what is in them), Holter Monitor reports, heart stress test results, EKG's, ER visit reports, hospitalizations, physical therapist reports, EMG's, CMAP, sleep studies, recording oximeter reports, and muscle biopsy report.

All testing results that "rule everything else out" and leave Periodic Paralysis as the only option need to be placed in the folder next. These include but are not limited to; lab reports, office notes (depending on what is in them), MRI's, spinal taps, brain scans, X-rays, EEG's, nerve conduction studies, colonoscopy, upper and lower GI's, neurological exams and much more.

A description of the symptoms, including paralytic episodes should be included, along with the list of triggers for those symptoms and the results of avoiding triggers or using medications or potassium. A disk with recordings of episodes could also fit in this section.

The daily vitals charts including potassium, oxygen, body temperature, glucose, blood pressure, heart rate, arrhythmia, oxygen levels and pH levels should also be included as well as surgeries, hospitalizations, ER visits, medication history and side effects and family medical history. All of these forms are found in this workbook.

With this book and all of your information in hand, you are prepared to "hit the doctors between the eyes with the facts." You are ready to receive a clinical diagnosis; one based on the facts, your symptoms and characteristics.

The Diagnosis

At the end of each appointment the doctor completes a form which is usually in tripilicate. The form has a large number of possible diseases or diagnoses listed with a number assigned to each. The diseases are categorized. These names and numbers are universal, used worldwide. They are the method for assigning a diagnosis and for billing insurance companies. By the end of the visit, several of the diseases may have been checked. This system is called the ICD-10 Codes Registry, (International Classification of Diseases).

To assist the doctor, an individual may offer the correct number for the Periodic Paralysis diagnosis. It has been assigned the number: G723 (G72.3) and is categorized as a disease of the nervous system and further sub-categorized as a disease of the myoneural junction (also known as neuromuscular) and muscle, although it is basically an ion channelopathy and a mineral metabolic disorder. Make sure to keep a copy of this form and it is prudent to also get a copy of the office notes.

Once the diagnosis is secure, the doctor will hopefully write a letter stating the diagnosis. It may contain the form or type of Periodic Paralysis, why and how the diagnosis was made, any recommendations, necessary instructions and explanations. A copy of this letter should be carried at all times.

The diagnosis and proper treatment of all the forms of Periodic Paralysis in a timely manner is absolutely imperative in order to avoid the possible complications including mitochondrial damage and autoimmune dysfunction and to slow or stop the progression of the disease, which can be permanent.

The Periodic Paralysis Guide And Workbook

The Future of Diagnosing Periodic Paralysis

As discussed in Chapter Five we have created a new, sensible, practical and more reliable way to diagnose Periodic Paralysis. This includes a checklist that contains the type of Periodic Paralysis based on the symptoms, degree of progression or 'level', and the 'stage' to which it has developed. It is our hope that doctors may review this form and use it in the near future, as the method to diagnose and understand the progression and stages of each individual's case of Periodic Paralysis.

A blank copy of this form, the instructions for how to complete it and a completed form are provided.

The Instructions:

The Number of Years Without a Diagnosis?
Age at diagnosis minus the age at the sign of the first symptom

Episodes of Paralysis or Muscle weakness?
Yes or No

Andersen-Tawil Syndrome Characteristics?
Yes or No

Form of Periodic Paralysis?
Based on Symptoms and Characteristics

Co-existing Conditions?
List and count then check the types: Autoimmune, Mitochondrial, Auto inflammatory or ?

Degree or Level of Progression?
Permanent muscle weakness? Exercise Intolerance? Permanent heart damage? Breathing muscle weakness? Other permanent Issues?
Check and count

Stage of Periodic Paralysis?
Stage One=periods of muscle weakness, or partial or full-body paralysis.
Stage Two=periods of muscle weakness, or partial or full-body paralysis and PP+ 1-10 (or more)
Stage Three= periods of muscle weakness, or partial or full-body paralysis and PP+ 1-10 (or more) and Autoimmune Dysfunction
Stage Four=periods of muscle weakness, or partial or full-body paralysis and PP+ 1-10 (or more) and Mitochondrial Dysfunction
Stage Five=periods of muscle weakness, or partial or full-body paralysis and PP+ 1-10 (or more) and Mitochondrial Dysfunction and Autoimmune Dysfunction

This formula is very clear to understand. It is sensible, practical and a more reliable way to diagnose Periodic Paralysis.

Get A Diagnosis

PPNI Periodic Paralysis Diagnosis Chart
Periodic Paralysis Plus 10 (or more) Syndrome (PP+10S)

Age **68** Age 1st Sign of PP **11** Age at Diagnosis **68** Yrs W/O Diagnosis **51**

Paralysis? Intermittent: Partial or (Full Paralysis) **✓**   Muscle Weakness **✓**
Gradual Muscle Weakness Only _____

ATS Characteristics:
Webbed 2-3 Toes, Curved little finger, Missing eye teeth and wisdom Teeth, Small mandible, low set ears, Long QT,

Types Periodic Paralysis:
HypoPP (Low Pot)_____ HyperPP (High Pot)_____ NormoPP (Normal Pot)_____
ATS (Low/High/Norm Pot + Long QT) **✓**   PMC (High Pot/Myotonia)_____
TPP (Low Pot/Thyroid)_____ Unknown_____

Co-existing Conditions:
Lactose Acidosis, Severe osteoporosis, Fibromyalgia, Type II Diabetes, Degenerative Disk Disease, Arthritis, Hiatal Hernia, Restless Leg Syndrome, Small Vessel Ischemia of the Brain, TIAs, Interstitial Cystitis, Dysautonomia, Allergies

Autoimmune **✓**   Mitochondrial **✓**   Other_____ Total # **13**

Degree of Progression:
Permanent Muscle Weakness **✓**   Exercise Intolerance **✓**
Permanent Heart Damage **✓**   Breathing muscle Weakness **✓**
Other Permanent Issues_____ Total # D of P **4**

Stages of Periodic Paralysis:
_____ Stage One=periods of muscle weakness, or partial or full-body paralysis.
_____ Stage Two=periods of muscle weakness, or partial or full-body paralysis and PP+ 1-10 (any number)
_____ Stage Three= periods of muscle weakness, or partial or full-body paralysis and PP+ 1-10 (any number) and Autoimmune Dysfunction
_____ Stage Four=periods of muscle weakness, or partial or full-body paralysis and PP+ 1-10 and Mitochondrial Dysfunction
✓ Stage Five=periods of muscle weakness, or partial or full-body paralysis and PP+ 1-10 and Mitochondrial Dysfunction and Autoimmune Dysfunction   Total Stage # **5**

Diagnosis: Type **ATS**   # of CC+ **13**   # of D of P **4**   Stage **5**

PPNI Periodic Paralysis Diagnosis Chart
Periodic Paralysis Plus 10 (or more) Syndrome (PP+10S)

Age_____ Age 1st Sign of PP_____ Age at Diagnosis_____ Yrs W/O Diagnosis_____

Paralysis?   Intermittent: Partial or Full Paralysis_____ Muscle Weakness_____

Gradual Muscle Weakness Only_____

ATS Characteristics:

_____

_____

Types Periodic Paralysis:

HypoPP (Low Pot)_____ HyperPP (High Pot)_____ NormoPP (Normal Pot)_____

ATS (Low/High/Norm Pot + Long QT)_____ PMC (High Pot/Myotonia)_____

TPP (Low Pot/Thyroid)_____ Unknown_____

Co-existing Conditions:

_____

_____

_____

_____

Autoimmune_____ Mitochondrial_____ Other_____ Total # _____

Degree of Progression:

Permanent Muscle Weakness_____ Exercise Intolerance_____

Permanent Heart Damage_____ Breathing muscle Weakness_____

Other Permanent Issues_____ Total # D of P_____

Stages of Periodic Paralysis:

_____Stage One=periods of muscle weakness, or partial or full-body paralysis.

_____Stage Two=periods of muscle weakness, or partial or full-body paralysis and PP+ 1-10 (any number)

_____Stage Three= periods of muscle weakness, or partial or full-body paralysis and PP+ 1-10 (any number) and Autoimmune Dysfunction

_____Stage Four=periods of muscle weakness, or partial or full-body paralysis and PP+ 1-10 and Mitochondrial Dysfunction

_____Stage Five=periods of muscle weakness, or partial or full-body paralysis and PP+ 1-10 and Mitochondrial Dysfunction and Autoimmune Dysfunction

Total Stage #_____

Diagnosis: Type _____ **# of CC+** _____ **# of D of P** _____ **Stage** _____

Periodic Paralysis Network, Inc. Sequim, Washington U.S.A. All rights reserved. Copyright © 2014

More about Diagnosing

Although I have refrained from editorializing in this book, some things still need to be said so, where appropriate, I have added a few articles I wrote which may need to be shared with medical professionals who lack proper understanding about Periodic Paralysis. Diagnosing is one of the areas that are discussed daily among individuals with Periodic Paralysis, as well as, the despicable treatment by the medical professionals in their lives.

After reading a post from one of the members of our PPNI Support, Education and Advocacy Group, I felt it was time to get on my soapbox and do a little editorializing again. It seems that doctors in general have learned little about Periodic Paralysis and even less about how to deal with chronically ill patients. They lack what is called "a good bedside manner." I wanted to take some time to put a doctor in his place and perhaps teach him a thing or two also. Because we are an advocacy group, as well as educational and supportive, I find I must advocate for our members safety, and well being. Therefore, I wrote the following:

Why Do You Need A Diagnosis?

"One of the members of our support group shared with us about another frustrating appointment with a "specialist" as she was attempting to get a diagnosis and proper treatment for her teenage daughter who has been suffering greatly during severe and painful episodes of paralysis several times a day and at night. The "specialist" in the process of being rude and arrogant, dared to ask the following question, "Why do you need a diagnosis?" and then made the statement "There is no treatment," not really expecting an answer or reply. Distressed and dismayed at yet another doctor's demeaning, dismissive and egotistical attitude and no diagnosis for her ill and suffering daughter, our member related the story to us on our PPN Support and Education Group.

In answer to the doctor's rhetorical question and ill-informed and unfortunate comment, Calvin responded with the following: "Why do you need a diagnosis?" Answer..."To stop the insanity and abuse they create by mistreating the condition. This phrase should be included as one of the triggers we use to find another doctor."

He is absolutely correct. The problem is individuals with Periodic Paralysis need a diagnosis. We need it for safety reasons in the doctors' office, the dentist office, an ambulance ride, the ER, the hospital, for surgeries and in any emergency. Most of us cannot take any drugs or medications due to idiosyncratic, paradoxical and iatrogenic effects nor can we have IV's because sodium and glucose can shift our potassium even lower and causes other life-threatening symptoms nor can we tolerate anesthesia due to possible malignant hyperthermia and/or more life-threatening arrhythmia, paralysis, possible cessation of breathing and death. We need a diagnosis so we can be safe and free from harm in any and all situations.

The medical professionals in our lives need to know that we have Periodic Paralysis and how to treat us or not treat us, as the case may be. They need to know that when we are in paralysis and struggling with arrhythmia, fluctuating blood pressure and heart rate, chocking, breathing issues and pain, that although we cannot open our eyes or speak, we can hear them. They need to know that we are not faking. We are not making it up.

Why would we?? Does anyone really think we want to be totally helpless and struggling for our life??

We also need a diagnosis to stop the constant, expensive and insane cycle of testing and retesting for every condition under the sun for an average of twenty years out of our life. (Some of our members did not get a diagnosis until they were in their eighth decade. I myself was diagnosed at the age of 62.) Because genetic testing is costly, narrow, biased and can only diagnose about half of all patients, diagnosing must be done clinically, based on symptoms, once "everything else is ruled out." REALLY?? How many medical conditions exist in which an individual intermittently has episodes of paralysis??

During the cycle of insanity for a diagnosis, drugs of every type are prescribed which are unnecessary and harmful causing more damage and possible death. New symptoms may develop and then more testing is done and new drugs prescribed. The insanity continues. Then comes the diagnosis of "conversion disorder" or "somatic symptoms." Psychotropic drugs are prescribed at this point. More damage is done and possible death may occur.

Without a diagnosis and proper treatment, the individual naturally becomes more ill because organs in the body are being damaged from the potassium shifting, exercise intolerance and gradual permanent muscle weakness sets in, heart problems get more severe, breathing muscles become affected, osteoporosis, kidney stones develop. Metabolic acidosis can kill us. Adaptive equipment like power wheelchairs and oxygen may be necessary. Without a diagnosis the patients will be unable to receive these much needed aides. Without a diagnosis, disability or social security is impossible to receive.

The child, teenager and young adult with Periodic Paralysis will need a diagnosis for appropriate treatment. He or she will need accommodations in school. Teachers and school nurses need to know how to deal with the symptoms and paralysis and understand what is happening and why. There may be a great deal of school missed. Sports and other activities need to be avoided. A special diet must be followed. Wheelchairs or other adaptive equipment may be needed. Without a diagnosis none of this will happen.

For the adult trying to support a family by holding down a job or a career and living with Periodic Paralysis without a diagnosis and proper treatment may lose their job. The years and years of medical testing, misdiagnosis, wrong medications, inappropriate treatment and more can result in financial ruin. This can lead to homes being lost, divorce may ensue, families will fall apart, friends back away, depression sets in and possible suicide may occur. A clear diagnosis and treatment may help others like employers, family members and friends to understand and be willing to help. Disability may be possible.

One of the most important results of a diagnosis for the individual with Periodic Paralysis and his or her family is validation. Validation that the illness does truly exist and that he or she is finally believed. They are vindicated. Vindicated of making it up, faking it or being a hypochondriac. They do not have "conversion disorder." They have been telling the truth.

And so doctor, "Why do we need a diagnosis?" We need a diagnosis because we want a chance at the quality of life you are experiencing. We need a diagnosis because we want to be treated with dignity and respect. We need a diagnosis because we want to be free of or ease our paralysis, arrhythmia, heart issues, breathing issues and more with the possibility of proper treatment or medication. We need a diagnosis because we would like to use our family's hard earned money to take care of our needs rather than paying for unnecessary testing and harmful drugs. We need a diagnosis so we can obtain adaptive equipment to make our lives and that of or loved ones easier. We need a diagnosis so we can be safe in emergency situations. We need a diagnosis because we want to live!!!

In conclusion, your rhetorical question and following comment indicate you lack any understanding of the ill patients who come to you for help. You obviously lack understanding, caring, compassion, empathy and sympathy. Your knowledge of Periodic Paralysis is obviously limited and based on archaic information because there is a great deal that can be done to treat our symptoms, once we have a diagnosis. You are obviously not living up to the Hippocratic oath that I assume you pledged early in your career. You are not doing the job for which you we hired. And you sir, are now fired!!!"

http://livingwithperiodicparalysis.blogspot.com/2014/09/why-do-you-need-diagnosis.html

Why haven't they done genetic testing?

This is another article related to diagnosing issues, which are misunderstood: One of our members was going through some medical testing working towards getting a concise and much needed diagnosis for Periodic Paralysis. The test measures nerve conduction and is predictably painful. The results may or may not detect Periodic Paralysis. As she was in tears and only half done with the testing, the doctor feeling sorry for her asked her asked, "Why haven't they done genetic testing?" He then decided not to complete the test, much to the relief of his patient. Though the doctor had the best of intentions, he did not understand the problem with seeking and receiving a concise diagnosis for one of the several known variants of Periodic Paralysis.

This is my response to the doctor:
"Why haven't they done genetic testing??" Really?? Maybe because it does not matter because only one half of us have a mutation that has been discovered and the testing at best is narrow and biased let alone expensive and virtually non-existent!! Genetic testing gives no guarantee for receiving a diagnosis. At this time, diagnosing for Periodic Paralysis must be based on an individual's symptoms and characteristics, depending on the type they have.

According to the American Heart Association, related to the study of genetics, the approach is complex and should include genome-wide studies, this is to rule out biased research and study. Also of note is that only one percent of human genome has been sequenced or transcribed into proteins. Therefore an enormous amount is yet to be learned about DNA.

This would indicate that genome-wide genetic testing would be the best way to test for the various forms of Periodic Paralysis, but since only one percent of human genome has actually been transcribed, it also indicates why more than half of those tested get negative results. The research labs run testing only for the tests requested by the doctors ordering them. If testing for only one form of Periodic Paralysis is requested, that is all that will be checked.

When genetic testing was being done and blood was sent overseas for testing for Periodic Paralysis, only the known mutations were searched for and they were either found or not found. There was no research done on what mutations on the same gene in the same exons or locations meant nor did they report those findings on the results if they were found in the denial letter sent to the individual. This is definite "bias" in the testing. One is left to believe there is no reason for their symptoms and to wonder about their own sanity. An individual's doctors, not understanding the above information, believe that the person does not have Periodic Paralysis.

Studies indicate that it takes an average of twenty years and is certainly very costly for someone with Periodic Paralysis to get a diagnosis. This is ludicrous and unconscionable. During those years an individual gets worse. They develop exercise intolerance, permanent muscle weakness, heart issues, breathing issues and are harmed from unnecessary medications. Some may even die.

Those twenty years or more consist of seeing doctor after doctor, specialist after specialist; taking test after test, because it is a condition in which a diagnosis is obtained by exclusion, it is diagnosed after everything else is ruled out.

Besides taking a long time it is very, very costly. I myself did not get a diagnosis until the age of 62. Some of our members in their eighth decade are still trying to get a diagnosis. Many die without a diagnosis, some very early in life, while trying to get a diagnosis. My own great uncle died at the age of 41 during an episode.

So, in conclusion, there is only a fifty percent chance that if an individual has genetic testing done a genetic mutation will be discovered. This chance reduces considerably when the testing done is biased and narrow. Whole genome testing by the correct and reputable lab may provide some answers but it is very expensive and most doctors will not order it nor will many medical insurance companies pay for it.

Periodic Paralysis needs to be diagnosed clinically, based on an individual's symptoms and characteristics.

http://livingwithperiodicparalysis.blogspot.com/2014/10/why-havent-they-done-genetic-testing.html

These articles may be copied and presented to medical professionals as needed. Many more articles about diagnosing can be found on the PPNI Blog.

Fourteen
Get Proper Medical Treatment
ASSEMBLE AND DIRECT THE TEAM

- ❖ **Getting Proper Treatment**
  - ➢ **Assemble a team of doctors (knowledgeable about PP or willing to learn).**
    - PCP
    - Neurologist
    - Electrocardiologist
    - Nephrologist
    - Endocrinologist
    - Counselor or therapist
    - Others as needed for symptoms
    - MDA doctors
  - ➢ **Direct the team**
    - Primary Care Doctor

The Plan

- ❖ Follow plan in Chapter Thirteen for securing a diagnosis, if needed.
- ❖ Make sure he or she has all of your medical records.
- ❖ Provide her with everything you can find written on Periodic Paralysis.
  - ➢ Keep up on the latest treatments.
    - Share with doctor.
- ❖ Follow the plans in Chapter Eleven as it applies to you.
  - ➢ Give a copy to your doctor.
- ❖ Ask for referrals as necessary in order to develop a "Team"
  - ➢ Neurologist
  - ➢ Electrocardiologist
  - ➢ Nephrologist
  - ➢ Endocrinologist
  - ➢ Physical therapist
  - ➢ Counselor or therapist
    - Have them write a letter stating you do not have a conversion disorder or are not faking it.
  - ➢ Others as needed for symptoms.
    - MDA doctors if possible.
      - Ask for a referral to your nearest MDA office
  - ➢ Contact your nearest MDA office to get a referral
    - BUT: Be very careful. (see Chapter Nine)
- ❖ Seek out Community Services
  - ➢ Transportation
  - ➢ Home Health Care

You are the leader of your medical team so it important for you to "hire" only doctors who will work with you and for you as you direct the team in your best interest.

Once you have found a caring doctor who is either knowledgeable about Periodic Paralysis or willing to learn about it and work with you, follow the plan in Chapter Thirteen for securing a diagnosis if needed.

If you already have a diagnosis, make sure the doctor has all of your medical records. Be sure to sign all release forms for each doctor you have seen, for all labs, tests of any kind, hospital visits, etc. for your new doctor. He or she will need all of your records, especially the ones, which include your diagnosis and lab work and testing which proves it. Use the ideas in Chapter Thirteen and the Personal Periodic Paralysis Journal in this book to help put it all together in a file. Add any and all new information as you get it. You may also gather your own records by going to the doctors, hospitals and labs yourself and collect the records for yourself and then pass them on to your doctor. This is the best way to ensure derogatory written records do not get passed from one doctor to another. It is important to take control over the accuracy of the information being shared about you.

Provide your doctor with all of the latest information you can find about Periodic Paralysis, especially about the type you have or believe you have. A copy of this book would also be helpful to share with him or her.

It is best to remember that doctors have very few treatment options for serious illness outside of administering pharmaceutical drugs or performing invasive surgeries. For individuals with Periodic Paralysis, this means there is little that they can do for those who cannot take medications or cannot have anesthesia for surgery. So it will be up to you to explain these things to the physicians and present them with your own plan. Follow the Plans from Chapter Eleven as it applies to your particular symptoms and type of Periodic Paralysis. You will need to experiment until you find what will work for you. Document your triggers, symptoms such as high or low blood pressure and oximeter readings, potassium meter readings, episodes of paralysis and how you are following the plan and share your progress with the doctor.

Ask for referrals as needed to specialists. Do not be afraid to ask. The most common ones needed may include a neurologist mostly to rule everything else out, but not needed after that; an electrocardiologist to treat the heart issues, especially the electrical issues which includes the arrhythmia and tachycardia or bradycardia; nephrologist if kidney issues are involved; endocrinologist who treat metabolic disorders of which Periodic Paralysis is; physical therapist who may be able to assess the muscle weakness and can order walkers, canes, wheelchairs, etc, as needed and a counselor or therapist to assist with the depression and anxiety, which may be involved. There may be other specialists necessary depending on the medical issues which develop such as a pulmonologist for breathing problems and the need for oxygen. Do not forget to get the records from each visit and all labs and tests and add these to your file.

You may also need home health care, respite, loaning of medical equipment or assistance with transportation, etc. so you may want to research the community services available for individuals who are disabled or seniors in your area. Have your doctor assist you with this. You may need referrals.

Get Proper Medical Treatment

Ask the primary care doctor to write letters, which state that you, in fact, have Periodic Paralysis. Ask the therapist or counselor to write a letter explaining that you do not have a conversion disorder. Use these letters when dealing with the specialists, paramedics if an ambulance must be called and emergency room (ER) staff in emergency situations.

Ask the doctors to assist with getting oxygen and equipment such as a blood sugar meter and strips, which can also be used with the cardy meter or ordering a cane, walker or wheelchair. Request a standing order for testing for metabolic acidosis, lactic acidosis and other possible complications.

Iatrogenic Medicine

Despite doing everything correctly to seek out and find a good and caring doctor and to get a diagnosis, we will still have occasion to be treated inappropriately, incorrectly, insufficiently, inadequately, inadvertently and adversely by the medical professionals we must deal with in order to treat the symptoms we experience. They just do not have the correct information, experience or training to deal with Periodic Paralysis.

The word "iatrogenic" refers to any type of inadvertent, adverse condition or illness, which is the result of a medical professional's activity, therapy or manner. This also refers to the inaction of a medical professional, which results in an adverse condition.

After researching the word, "iatrogenic," I believe that most of those individuals with Periodic Paralysis have been on the receiving end of this, especially the wrong diagnoses we have received and the wrong administration of drugs for wrongly diagnosed conditions. Also, by the administration of certain drugs for our condition that are harming us by causing kidney stones and metabolic acidosis and even death in a few cases. This is usually inadvertent (not on purpose, of course, in most cases).

Since so little is known about Periodic Paralysis, we need to be our own experts about our own bodies and our own disease!! If you are on any medications, regardless of the fact they may be for your particular form of PP, please study it thoroughly. That includes the use of anesthesia. If you do not study it by really digging and searching for "RARE" side effects or go to a website where people are suing over the use of a drug to discover these things, they can be overlooked by the doctors or yourself.

I know of a few cases recently among members of our boards in which, certain anesthesia thought to be permissible for someone with ATS, a form of PP, turned out to possibly cause long QT heartbeats and other cardiac issues, muscle weakness and respiratory issues. One member was in the hospital for almost a month, after a procedure, due to those side effects and issues. This was a definite "iatrogenic" result. After researching it as described above, I found the hidden information.

I believe that this new word, "iatrogenic," also can apply to those individuals with Periodic Paralysis who become more ill due to the lack of a diagnosis. Many of our members have been waiting years for a diagnosis. (I was not diagnosed until the age of 62.) Most doctors are reluctant to diagnose the various forms of Periodic Paralysis although everything else has been ruled out. They insist that a patient must have a genetic code found during DNA testing. The problem with this ideation is that nearly half of all people with Periodic Paralysis have no known genetic code discovered yet and may never have in their lifetime. So it must be diagnosed based on symptoms and characteristics. This is called a clinical diagnosis, the manner in which most diseases are diagnosed.

So if doctors are withholding a diagnosis or failing to diagnose due to out of date information or a lack of proper understanding and knowledge of the disease and thus patients are not getting proper treatment, these individuals are becoming more ill and or dying due to "iatrogenic" medical treatment.

Our PPNI Forum is designed to educate everyone on how to better understand Periodic Paralysis. We are searching everyday for better answers to our questions and our needs. We place the information we discover on the boards everyday. It is up to each individuals to decide how to use it. We must all make decisions about how to deal with our symptoms and conditions, but we must make "educated" decisions. It seems we cannot simply follow the lead of our doctors. In most cases we know more than they do about Periodic Paralysis and how it affects us. So those of us with Periodic Paralysis must be our own best experts with our disease, because no one else is watching out for us.

As the co-founders and co-directors the Periodic Paralysis Network, Inc. we work towards the improvement of the quality and safety of patients from all over the world with the various forms of Periodic Paralysis, which we know is very rare, inherited, disabling mineral metabolic disorder. Our focus is on educational resources to build self-reliance and self-empowerment and to prevent possible harm from improper treatment. Our approach to treatment focuses on the self-monitoring of vitals and the management of symptoms through natural methods. We also offer strategies to understanding the disease, getting a proper diagnosis, managing the symptoms, and assisting caregivers and family members. We are patient-safety-related due to the serious nature and potential life-threatening symptoms and side effects of this condition if it is not treated correctly.

Conclusion

As we are all aware, very few of us will get any real help from a doctor even if we find one who knows about the disease and is kind, sympathetic and empathetic. This is due to the fact that most of us are unable to tolerate the known medications and the doctors do not know how to help us.

So, although I have a primary care physician and several good specialists, Calvin and I are still left to deal with my episodes of paralysis and my other symptoms with no real help from the medical field. They do not know how to help me, but treat me well and look after the things they can; like my heart problems, power wheelchair, oxygen, diabetes strips and labs. I appreciate and understand their lack of knowledge of such a rare and baffling disease. My doctors trust us with the plan we have created after much research and trial and error.

In order to get the best medical treatment we can, we need to be our own experts about our own bodies and our own disease and we must teach and train the medical professionals we see.

Fifteen
Direct The Paramedics And EMT's
NO IV PLEASE

- > Direct the team
  - Paramedics and EMT's

Introduction

Remember that you are the team leader, receiving and directing one's proper medical treatment does not stop at the doctor's office door. Individuals with Periodic Paralysis find themselves dealing with paramedics and EMT's many times before and after finally getting a diagnosis. It is essential that you be able to direct the team that will appear at your door ready to hook you up to an IV or the team at the hospital ready to take your blood and to give you medications.

The best way to do that is to prepare ahead of time for medical emergencies.

- ❖ Call and set up an appointment to meet with your local paramedics, nearest Ambulance Company or fire department to discuss your particular situation.
  - > Provide them with as much information as possible about your type of Periodic Paralysis
  - > Provide them with information from your file folder.
  - > Give them a copy of this or our other book about Periodic Paralysis
  - > If you live alone give them a key to your home or let them know where a key is to get in to help you.
- ❖ At home put the emergency list on a bulletin board or refrigerator.
- ❖ Carry copies of all the information with you at all times.
  - > In folder.
  - > In purse, wallet.
  - > In medic alert bracelet.
  - > In car glove box.
  - > Pin to car visor.
  - > In badge holders, attached to chain around neck.
- ❖ Know when to call an ambulance.
  - > No tourniquet
  - > No IV

Meeting with your local paramedics is probably the best way to begin preparing for medical emergencies. It may take a few phone calls to discover which are the correct fire department and/or ambulance company for your neighborhood. Set up an appointment or discuss your issues with the chief paramedic or fire chief over the phone.

Provide them with as much information as possible about your type of Periodic Paralysis or the type you believe you have. Provide them with information on how to treat you. Be sure to include a list of the medications you cannot have. Give them copies of all of your important medical information. Make sure to give them copies of the letters written by your doctor or counselor backing up your diagnosis or possible diagnosis and information indicating you do not have a conversion disorder and that you are not a malingerer. If you live alone, be sure to either give them a key to your house or let them know where one will be in an emergency. Providing them with a copy of this book or our first one may be a good idea.

Since the paramedics may not have had any training about your condition or new ones may show up or in case they have forgotten, making an emergency list of the things the paramedics need to know as soon as they enter your door is the single most important thing you can do. It needs to be posted on a bulletin board or on the refrigerator in plain view. Although you may have a spouse, friend or family member there with you, you may not be able to speak and those with you may forget to relay important information. Having it written down and posted will be helpful for everyone involved.

As suggested previously, you should have a folder with your entire collection of medical information and information about Periodic Paralysis. The emergency list should also be in the file, on the top. The folder should be in an obvious and easily accessible place known to everyone in the family. A copy of this book should be part of the collection.

Making several copies of this information and carrying a set with you would be a good idea. You may end up in an emergency somewhere out of your home and paramedics may arrive who will know nothing about you. If carrying your entire file with you is not practical, then make sure to at least have your emergency list handy. You can carry your medical information or the emergency list with you in several ways: in a folder, in a purse or wallet, in a medic alert bracelet, in a car glove box, pinned to the car visor or in a badge holder attached to a chain bracelet secured around your neck. You need to be creative but also realistic. Be sure it is in an obvious and easily seen place.

When making the emergency list, remember that you may be alone and may not be able to speak. Think of the things they will need to know. First, they cannot put you on a glucose or sodium IV. If they take a blood sample, they cannot use a tourniquet because it can make the potassium levels appear higher than they are.

The key to being safe and receiving appropriate treatment by the paramedics is to be prepared ahead of time.

http://livingwithperiodicparalysis.blogspot.com/2013/12/periodic-paralysis-and-erthe-narrative.html
http://livingwithperiodicparalysis.blogspot.com/2013/12/avoiding-pitfalls-of-emergency-room.html

Direct The Paramedics And EMT's

Emergency Chart

My name is Susan. I am 66 years old and I have a very rare disease called Period Paralysis. The type I have is Andersen-Tawil Syndrome.

Potassium shifts in my body if I am hypokalemic, hyperkalemic or normokalemic. I become totally paralyzed when the potassium shifts from my organs and goes into my muscles. I am unable to move in any way and am not able to speak or open my eyes. I look like I am asleep, **BUT**, I can hear everything going on around me. I can hear everything being said.

I may be able to move my index finger on my right hand. If you ask "yes" or "no" questions, I may be able to answer. Up and down is "yes" and sideways is "no".

My husband, Calvin, knows exactly what to do for me, so listen carefully to what he says and follow his directions. If he is not with me or is unable to speak or help me please follow the outline below:

If I must go to a hospital take me to Valley Medical Center. My doctors are:

1. Dr. A   PCP   360-000-0000
2. Dr. B   Cardiologist   360-000-0000
3. Dr. C   Renal Specialist   360-000-0000
4. Dr. D   Endocrinologist   360-000-0000

- Please talk to me and tell me what you are doing to me and for me.
- Please make sure I am comfortable.
- Please make sure I am reclining but not lying flat.
- Please be sure my oxygen is on and working.
- Please cover me with a light sheet or blanket because I get cold.
- Please make sure my head and neck are supported. My head will fall to the side and can hurt a great deal.
- Please do not try to move me when I am paralyzed. Damage can occur to my muscles and joints.
- Please do not put me on an IV. I cannot have saline or glucose…if one must be used, mannitol may be ok.
- Please do not give me any medications of any kind to include antibiotics.
- Please do not give me any type of anesthesia, to include lidocaine.
- Please do not use a tourniquet if blood is to be taken to check my potassium levels.
- Please do not put any food or liquid in my mouth, I will choke because I cannot swallow.
- Please watch my breathing it may stop or be very shallow.
- Please watch my swallowing. I may choke.
- Please monitor my heart. I have a heart loop monitor in my chest. I have long QT interval beats, arrhythmias, tachycardia, bradycardia and my heart may stop beating. I may go into cardiac arrest.
- Please do not be alarmed if I have myoclonic jerks or fasciculations. It may mean that I am hyperkalemic, and is not a seizure.
- Please have patience. I will come out of it eventually. It may last 15 minutes to several hours or I may go in and out of it.
- Please be ready with a bedpan or be ready to help me to the bathroom. I will have to urinate urgently after I come out of it but will still be too weak to walk by myself to the bathroom.

Other conditions: Hyperkalemic Periodic Paralysis/Paramyotonia Congenita (genetic); type II diabetes; fibromyalgia; severe osteoporosis (bone crush of spine); heart arrhythmia: PVC's, PAC's PJC's, errants, ST segment abnormalities, long QT interval heartbeat, non-conducted PAC's, abnormal T waves and angina; exercise intolerance; small vessel ischemia of the brain; degenerative disk disease; diverticulitis; arthritis of the spine; acid reflux; hiatal hernia; high cholesterol/triglycerides; restless leg syndrome; muscle myopathy; interstitial cystitis; prolapsed bladder; dysautonomia.

My Medications: None, Oxygen Therapy 2liters 24/7

Susan Quentine Knittle-Hunter   Born January 00, 1900
000 Summer Road
Small Town, Anywhere 12345   1-000-000-0000   Emergency: Husband: Calvin Hunter: 1-000-000-0000

http://livingwithperiodicparalysis.blogspot.com/2013/11/emergency-instruction-chart-november-19.html
http://livingwithperiodicparalysis.blogspot.com/2013/12/when-to-call-for-ambulance-december-3.html

When to Call an Ambulance

After experiencing and studying Periodic Paralysis and Andersen-Tawil Syndrome, I have learned that an ambulance does not need to be called every time I become paralyzed. When I have a paralytic episode, I will usually be better within a few hours. For most individuals with Periodic Paralysis, this is the case.

It may be necessary, however, to call 911 or go to the ER if difficulties develop with breathing, the heart or with choking or swallowing regardless of the form of Periodic Paralysis an individual has.

However, when dealing with hypokalemia, moderately low levels of potassium, below 2.5, may create the following serious issues and may need emergency care: exceptionally high blood pressure, rapid or irregular heart beat, low oxygen, signs of metabolic acidosis, seizures and dark urine.

When dealing with hyperkalemia, high levels of potassium, the following may be helpful to be aware of: if the level is 6.0 or more than emergency treatment may be necessary. Call 911 or go to the emergency room if the heartbeat is weak or absent, blood pressure is seriously low, or there is a change in breathing, nausea or loss of consciousness. Mild hypervenatlation accompanying hyperkalemia may be due to metabolic acidosis and may need emergency treatment.

If an individual has Andersen-Tawil Syndrome (ATS), they experience episodes of paralysis based on low or high potassium levels or there may be episodes in normal ranges. Those with ATS experience serious ventricular arrhythmia with the possibility of life-threatening long QT interval heartbeats. They must be monitored closely. They may experience any of the above symptoms, especially, trouble with breathing, with the heart or with choking or swallowing. If these occur then an ambulance may be necessary.

When dealing with Normokalemic Periodic Paralysis, any of the above symptoms may develop and may need observing or emergency care, despite the potassium level.

It is imperative for one with Periodic Paralysis, and those close to him or her, to know what is 'normal' for their own symptoms. It is also important to know and understand the above information. An emergency chart and all medical information should be handy in case an ambulance must be called. I keep this information in a plastic folder along with everything I know is important and that the paramedics and EMT's must know when coming to my aid in an emergency and for the doctors when I get to the hospital. I approach it as if I will have no one with me to explain my needs. I keep it near the door and take it with me when I leave home.

I want to add here, that an important reason for going to the ER, if a person does not have a diagnosis, is to get the attacks documented, a "paper trail" is often needed. Proof of the episodes must be established.

Sixteen
Direct The ER And Hospital Staff
AVOID THE PITFALLS

- **Direct the team.**
  - **Emergency rooms**
  - **Hospital staff**

Introduction

It is important to be prepared before an ambulance team appears at the door ready to attach an IV to someone with Periodic Paralysis. In most emergencies the patient will be transported in the ambulance to the hospital and be seen, evaluated and treated in the emergency room and possibly be admitted to the hospital if the situation is serious enough. Just as it is important to be prepared for the paramedics, it is equally important to be prepared for the emergency room and to be able to deal with and direct the staff for the best and safest treatment possible.

The following plan is in an outline form for easier understanding and to use as a checklist.

- ❖ Call hospital administration office
  - ➢ Explain your problem
    - Tell them the history of visits and the problems during them
    - Tell them about your fears due to the previous visits
    - Explain your diagnosis or possible diagnosis
    - Explain your plan to bring in all your records for your file
    - Ask how you can speak to the supervisor of the ER
- ❖ Call the ER supervisor or make an appointment to meet with him/her
  - ➢ Explain your problem
    - Tell them the history of visits and the problems during them
    - Tell them about your fears due to the previous visits
    - Explain your diagnosis or possible diagnosis
    - Explain your plan to bring in all your records for your file
- ❖ Meet with ER supervisor or representative in person
  - ➢ Bring your significant other or a friend or family member
  - ➢ Present your
    - Records
    - Name and numbers of your doctors
    - Information about Periodic Paralysis
    - Your personal emergency chart
  - ➢ Bring this book or our other book
  - ➢ Bring copied from the internet
    - The types
      - Andersen-Tawil Syndrome?
      - Hypokalemic Periodic Paralysis?
      - Hyperkalemic Periodic Paralysis?
      - How to take your labs (no tourniquet)

- How to treat your symptoms
- How to diagnose, if not done yet
- ❖ Your diagnosis reports (from doctors) if you have them
- ❖ List of medications you cannot have
  - ➢ No IVs
  - ➢ No medications that paralyze
  - ➢ No meds that cause long QT (if it applies)
- ❖ List of medications you take
- ❖ List of other medical issues
  - ➢ Possibly diabetes, heart problems, etc
- ❖ Records of previous labs and tests which helped with the diagnosis or ruled other things out to include but not limited to:
  - ➢ EKG's
  - ➢ Holter monitors results
  - ➢ EMG's
  - ➢ EEG's
  - ➢ Muscle biopsy
  - ➢ Sleep studies
  - ➢ Pulmonary study
  - ➢ Physical therapy
- ❖ Letter from therapist clearing you of mental issues
  - ➢ Good to be seeing a therapist to help deal with
    - Failing health
    - Moral support
- ❖ Possibly a standing prescription from your doctor:
  - ➢ "if muscle weakness or paralysis"
    - "Blood serum labs for potassium"
- ❖ Have hospital records copied by:
  - ➢ Records department or
  - ➢ ER personnel
  - ➢ Explain anything else you believe is important

The Emergency Room and Hospital: Our Greatest Fear

Although individuals who have Periodic Paralysis are extremely ill, face serious medical issues and should be closely followed by medical professionals as well as face emergency situations daily, many avoid calling an ambulance and being seen in an ER or being hospitalized. It is the biggest concern discussed in the discussion groups.

The stories are endless and nearly daily another new member relates a horrifying story of frightening, unconscionable, ignorant, negligent, bullying, arrogant, disbelieving, harmful, hurtful, inexcusable, forceful, life threatening, disgusting, unbelievable, horrible, demeaning, abominable, offensive, appalling, and shameful treatment at the hands of the medical professionals they encounter in an ambulance, emergency room and hospital. They tell of being ignored, scoffed at, laughed at, lied about, lied too, improperly medicated, pinched, hit, misdiagnosed, accused of drinking or drug abuse, given diagnoses of mental illness or demanded to sit up, stand up or to move in some way when they are in paralysis. Others tell of being put on an IV or medication and being made worse, harmed or nearly killed. Still others tell us of family members who have died do to the improper treatment in the ER or hospital or by the provoking of symptoms in order to diagnosis the person.

We are living in the year 2014, nearly 2015, not the dark ages. No one should have to endure the effects of the wrong medications or treatments from the medical professionals whom we seek out for help in the ER or hospital. All medical professionals need to be trained about Periodic Paralysis and the correct ways to recognize the symptoms and to treat appropriately and at the very least, **LISTEN** to patients with Periodic Paralysis when in need of medical assistance. No one with any form of Periodic Paralysis should be forced into full-body paralysis and pain, heart arrhythmia, blood pressure fluctuation, choking, damage to his or her organs and the risk of possible death from a forced IV or medication. No one should have to experience more stress in such a situation, which, makes the makes the attack worse, and the fear of dying while unable to move in any way or cry out for help. This is archaic, inexcusable and unconscionable.

Hopefully, through awareness by planning ahead and following the plan for directing the ER and hospital staff will begin to change the way people with Periodic Paralysis are treated.

Avoid the Pitfalls

In order to avoid the pitfalls of the emergency room and to be certain to get the best and safest treatment when arriving at the hospital, it is necessary to be prepared in advance. This is much the same way as preparing for the paramedics but more detailed. The hospital will require much more information.

Research your nearest hospital with an emergency room, the one you will be taken to if an ambulance is called to your home. Contact the administration office. Tell your story, about your previous visits or problems if there were any, your fears and why. Explain your diagnosis or suspected diagnosis and why it is suspected. Explain your plan to share your medical records. Ask how they would like this to be done. They may ask them to be mailed or hand carried. Then ask for the best way to contact the ER supervisor in person.

Speak with the supervisor of the ER. Repeat your previous conversation with the administrator. Then set up a meeting, if possible. At the meeting present him or her with your complete file, journal with everything listed in the outline and a copy of this book, if possible. Bring copies of everything you have collected about your form of Periodic Paralysis. Answer any and all questions. One cannot be too prepared for an emergency.

The Plan in Action

Personally, after experiencing all of the treatment described, I refused to go to the ER and Calvin refused to let me go to or stay in a hospital. However, two years ago, Calvin and I moved to a new home in another state. I immediately called the nearest fire department and hospital. I explained my medical issues. The fire chief took notes and the hospital asked me to bring in my records to have them be put in the system. I did just that.

While there, I explained that they have to monitor my breathing; make sure I do not choke and monitor my heart due to the tachycardia, and arrhythmia, watching especially for the long QT interval heartbeat. They are not to hook me to an IV and not to give me glucose or any medications. They are not to use a tourniquet or have me make a fist if they need to take my blood. They should look through my file and folder for any other information they may need. It is also important for them to know to listen to your significant other (if you are lucky enough to have one), who will be your voice, if you cannot speak or explain things to them.

About a year ago, this was all put to the test when I had a possible small stroke (TIA). Calvin called 911 and my doctor. She called the hospital ER and told them about my condition (Andersen-Tawil Syndrome). When the paramedics arrived, Calvin handed each of them my emergency chart with instructions. They read them, asked a few questions and got to work checking my vitals and getting me ready to transport to the hospital. With Calvin's coaching, they followed every detail and I was safely taken to the ER. Upon arriving, the same thing happened. More copies were made of my emergency chart and the doctors referred to my medical records already in the system. They were very careful with everything they did or did not do to me or for me.

Calvin and I were very happy and relieved. They believed us and followed our instructions. We no longer fear a trip to the ER. I have no concerns about any future trips in an ambulance to the ER or if I need to be hospitalized. All of our preparation was worth it for peace of mind and the knowledge that I will be safe and properly cared for in the event of future emergencies.

http://livingwithperiodicparalysis.blogspot.com/2013/12/periodic-paralysis-and-erthe-narrative.html
http://livingwithperiodicparalysis.blogspot.com/2013/12/avoiding-pitfalls-of-emergency-room.html
http://livingwithperiodicparalysis.blogspot.com/2013/12/periodic-paralysis-and-erthe-narrative.html
http://livingwithperiodicparalysis.blogspot.com/2013/12/avoiding-pitfalls-of-emergency-room.html

Seventeen
Prognosis
THE BEST YOU CAN BE

As written in our previous book, when I realized that I had Periodic Paralysis, I wanted to know what to expect. How long will I live? How bad will I get? Can this disease be reversed if I get proper treatment? Will I lose my ability to walk? Will I ever drive again? Will I need to be in an assisted living program? Is there medication to stop the total paralytic episodes? What are my chances of dying from the long QT interval heart beat? Will my breathing continue to get more difficult until I can no longer breathe on my own? Is there any medication I can take if I get another bladder infection? What happens if I need an operation and cannot use anesthetics? What can I do to stop the pain in my shoulder and back since I cannot take any pain medications? When I go into cardiac arrest, is it worth trying to save me? Will I end up on dialysis due to kidney failure? Can I travel? What will happen if I end up in the Emergency Room again and they cannot help me with any medications?

My research to answer these questions, led me to an inadequate amount of information; both in the number of articles and the amount written. I found only a few short blurbs. These passages were and are copied over and over on the different websites related to the condition. Most are simply written by professional people who have no form of Periodic Paralysis and no real understanding of the disease. As well as being short and lacking information, I find the content to be simply misleading such as indicating that muscle damage can be reversed and that most people do well on medication. The specialists in the field write little more of what to expect in the studies of and articles about Periodic Paralysis. It seems strange that a disease as serious and as complex as Periodic Paralysis has only two or three short and misleading sentences written about what to expect for the rest of our lives!

Since writing the above paragraphs and after researching, studying, managing a forum and support group for individuals with all forms of Periodic Paralysis, discussing all aspects of it every day for nearly four years, writing a blog and two books about it, following the plan and ideas in this book and continuing to live four years after almost dying, I have learned that there are many answers to each question and for each person. There are no absolutes.

For many people with Periodic Paralysis their life span will be normal with very mild symptoms, but for others there may be severe complications and their life may be shortened. For some individuals with Periodic Paralysis, an off label drug may can control the symptoms. For others, however, they are not without side effects. For many more individuals the drugs do not work. For most people with Periodic Paralysis the weakness and paralysis are intermittent. There is a beginning and end and between the episodes the individual is normal. Some of these individuals can lead a fairly normal life. However, for many individuals the quality of life is compromised and the weakness can linger or become permanent. Some of them will become disabled and debilitated, require the use of a power wheelchair and will probably be unable to work a job or have a career. In some rare cases, Periodic Paralysis can cause death.

The good news is that for most individuals the paralysis and symptoms can be controlled using natural and common sense methods. Each individual with Periodic Paralysis has the opportunity to be the best they can be by individualizing their own plan based on the ideas in this book.

Eighteen
The Conclusion
HOPE

I would like to conclude this book with what was originally written to be the preface for this book. The narration is one of **hope**, and I decided I wanted to conclude this guide and workbook with this most important message.

A preface for a book is written to explain what the book is about, why the author wrote the book, why it is important, where the idea for the book originated, how it came to be and how long it took to write. With this in mind, I will begin by saying that this book is about a very rare, hereditary, and debilitating mineral metabolic disorder, with which I have been diagnosed, called Periodic Paralysis. My husband Calvin and I previously wrote one book about this subject, *living with Periodic Paralysis: The Mystery Unraveled,* in which we provide **hope** to others by telling our story, providing information about Periodic Paralysis not found anywhere else, providing information about how to better manage symptoms and the psychological and social aspects of living with the condition. I felt the need, however, to write an addendum, a user-friendly workbook and guide to assist individuals with this condition to be the best they can be by using the natural and common sense methods as outlined in the first book. This is important because very little information exists about how to treat the symptoms of Periodic Paralysis, other than the use of off label drugs, which can be harmful to many individuals or are not tolerated well. The idea for this book originated from my own experiences, study and experimentation and took more than four years to write. Our story of **hope** is related in the following paragraphs.

We now know I have more than one form of Periodic Paralysis, which is a very rare, debilitating, metabolic disorder. After my diagnosis in 2011 at the age of 62, many doctors, including the specialists, told me that there is nothing they can do for me. I can take no medications nor can I have any type of surgery. I was dying from the lifelong effects of the condition and the wrong treatment and drugs I had been given over the years. After hearing this, the only thing my husband, Calvin, had nearly four years ago was **hope** and determination and a will to find a way to save my life. I would be dead now if it were not for his persistent research and fight for the things that now keep me alive and are giving me a better quality of life. He found that preparing and feeding me a pH balanced diet with needed supplements, providing me with oxygen therapy, helping me to discover and avoid my triggers, sheltering me from stress, keeping me hydrated, monitoring my vitals and remaining optimistic brought me back from the brink of death and reduced my paralytic episodes from four or five full body attacks a day lasting several hours at a time, to one every two or three months!

Calvin had **hope**. He had a desire that things would turn out for the best. He was correct in what he did and how he did it and was optimistic that I would get better. He maintained **hope** that I would improve in all ways and the truth is that I did. Since that time, because of his **hope**, determination and optimism, together we wrote and published our first book about Periodic Paralysis in May of 2013, *living with Periodic Paralysis: The Mystery Unraveled.* It is about how he maintained **hope** and brought me back from near death, to be well enough to write a book about it and to share our discoveries with others.

Now that we have written one book about Periodic Paralysis why would we need to write another? The reason is the same as for the first book. We know there is a need, a real necessity, for a second book about Periodic Paralysis. We needed to create a user-friendly tool or workbook, which would help individuals with Periodic Paralysis to carry out the plans and ideas in the first book in order to be the best they can be by natural means. We needed to give them **hope**.

We know this because we deal daily with over 300 very ill individuals, from around the world, in our Periodic Paralysis Network Support, Education and Advocacy Group and others who contact me by email through our PPN Website, our PPN Facebook Pages, our PPN Blog or through searching for us after reading our first book. They are attempting to find the names of specialists who can help them and diagnose them and seeking a simple pill or medication to stop the paralysis and other cruel 'quality of life stealing' symptoms plaguing them daily. These individuals, their families and caregivers, and several new members each week, need **hope** and we spend our days providing support, education, advocacy, validation and **hope** in an otherwise hopeless world for them.

The truth is there are very few "specialists" or doctors in the world who know about or fully understand all aspects of the many forms of Periodic Paralysis. There is no simple pill or drug; no magic cure for Periodic Paralysis. There are only off-label drugs, which are helpful for some members with certain forms of Periodic Paralysis, but they have serious side affects. Many individuals cannot tolerate them or must stop taking them after the side affects like metabolic acidosis, osteoporosis, or kidney stones develop. Most doctors do not recognize Periodic Paralysis and genetic testing is nearly non-existent for most forms and therefore they will not diagnose their patients or will diagnose them with somatic disorders. However, when these individuals come to our forum, we are able to provide them with **hope.**

Hope is a sense of wanting a thing to be true or for it to happen and having faith that it is likely or possible. **Hope** is a feeling or a wish that situations or things will result in what is best. We provide this for our members. We provide **hope** and methods to assist them to find a doctor who cares and to get a diagnosis based on their symptoms. We provide **hope** and methods to assist them to relieve their symptoms in natural ways. We have **hope** that individuals with various forms of Periodic Paralysis will be able to improve their lives with the information and methods we have learned and I practice everyday and share in this second user friendly book which is a guide, a handbook, a journal, a series of life changing plans made up of goals and objectives and a workbook. *The Periodic Paralysis Guide and Workbook: Be The Best You Can Be Naturally*, offers **HOPE** to everyone with Periodic Paralysis, in the same manner as our book, *living with Periodic Paralysis: The Mystery Unraveled.*

We have been formulating and writing this workbook, since before we completed writing and publishing our first book in May of 2013. We envisioned a personalized book to accompany the first book. We envisioned a handbook that could be carried with individuals, who have all forms of Periodic Paralysis, to their doctor appointments, the ER and the hospital, which contained the information their doctors would need to treat them and diagnose them. We envisioned a guide with the goals and objectives of the plans in

The Conclusion

the first book expanded as well as the simple instructions to carry them out. We envisioned a workbook to include more charts, forms and a medical journal to individualize and complete in the book itself. We envisioned all of this and all of the information provided in our blog, on our website and shared and discussed in our support group in one handy book. We envisioned more explanation; information and more specific detail to help guide individuals to better health and to be the best they can be through natural means in a user-friendly manner. Our new workbook is this vision, which has become a reality.

As written in our first book, *"We **hope** everyone reading this book will have a better understanding of Periodic Paralysis. If you have a form of Periodic Paralysis, we **hope** you can improve the quality of your life by following our natural and common sense plans and advice. If you do not have a diagnosis we **hope** our ideas will be instrumental in helping you to get a diagnosis. If you are a doctor or health care provider, we **hope** you will be able to recognize, diagnose and treat individuals with Periodic Paralysis correctly, in a timely manner. If you are a social worker, therapist, caregiver, family member or friend, we **hope** you will be able to offer the understanding and support needed to your patient, family member, or friend who has this condition with your newly gained information. We especially **hope** you will know that you are not alone."*

In conclusion, we have **hope** and are optimistic that some individuals can tolerate the off-label drugs available and maintain a productive life. However, as mentioned previously, we know that many individuals with Periodic Paralysis cannot handle the effects of those drugs. They are worsened by them or do not respond well to them and we know that even though some members are taking the drugs, they continue to have symptoms and paralysis. We remain **hopeful** that they can follow the plans laid out in our book, improve their conditions and live a much more normal and productive life. We remain **hopeful** and optimistic because we see it happening everyday for the members of our Periodic Paralysis Network (PPNI) Support, Education and Advocacy Group and to those who are reading our first book. We share our knowledge and experience and everyday we see and hear about the lives being changed for those who are willing to make the lifestyle changes. It is not an easy path for us. We must walk a constant tightrope, but we do not give up **hope**.

We may not be able to provide anyone who has Periodic Paralysis with a cure or a magic drug or a diagnosis or a specialist who can help them, but we do know that through this user-friendly workbook we can give others **hope** through the knowledge we share, the ideas we pass along in all areas of dealing with and managing their symptoms and with validation and support. We wrote this, the second book about Periodic Paralysis, to give **hope** to others who suffer with this condition and to guide them to be the best they can be naturally.

Section III
The Journal

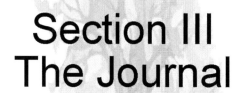

Nineteen
The Personal Periodic Paralysis Journal
PUT IT ALL TOGETHER

The following medical journal was created and designed to include every aspect of an individual's medical history in order to present a full and complete picture of the process and progress of this condition for diagnosis and treatment. It covers the following areas: personal medical history, medical testing history, medication history, patient Periodic Paralysis symptoms and characteristics and family medical history and much more. Every issue covered in this book has a form, chart, graph, table, outline or page included and may be copied or completed in this workbook and may be completed as necessary or desired. It is meant to be totally individualized and to fit each individual's needs.

The Personal Periodic Paralysis Journal

Name _____ Date_____

Date of Birth_____ M_____F_____

Address_____

_____

Phone Numbers (Home)_____(Cell)_____

Insurance Company_____

Insurance Numbers _____

Height _____Weight _____Blood Type_____

Type Of Periodic Paralysis _____

Diagnosis: Genetic _____ Clinical _____ No Diagnosis_____

Date Of Diagnosis _____

Name Of Diagnosing Doctor _____

Suspected diagnosis (if no diagnosis) _____

First symptom and age _____

_____

The Personal Periodic Paralysis Journal

History Of Diagnosis

If you have a diagnosis, how long did it take you to get, from onset of symptoms?
_____
_____
_____
_____
_____
_____

What type of doctor diagnosed you?
_____
_____
_____

If you do not have a diagnosis, how long have you been waiting for a diagnosis?
_____
_____
_____

Why won't the doctor diagnose you?
_____
_____
_____
_____

If you had a clinical diagnosis and a "Periodic Paralysis Specialist" took away your diagnosis, please explain why.
_____
_____
_____
_____

Was the "specialist" an MDA doctor? _____ An ATS specialist? _____

A PP specialist? _____ A neurologist? _____ Other? _____

Were you denied a diagnosis because you had other conditions co-existing with your Periodic Paralysis symptoms?
_____

Has everything else been ruled out? _____

Are you trying to find a doctor to diagnose you? _____

Description Of Episodes Of Paralysis

Average length of time for episodes?
Caused by: Low potassium? High potassium? Normal potassium?
Potassium and/or other medications or methods used to stop an episode:

_____
_____
_____
_____
_____
_____
_____
_____
_____
_____
_____
_____
_____
_____
_____
_____
_____
_____
_____
_____
_____
_____
_____
_____
_____
_____
_____
_____
_____
_____
_____
_____
_____
_____
_____

The Personal Periodic Paralysis Journal

Description Of Symptoms
Before, During And After Episodes

The Personal Periodic Paralysis Journal

Symptoms Of HypoPP, NormoPP And ATS (Ttypically)

(circle or check those that apply)

Muscles
Fatigue
Pain in the joints
Muscle weakness
Muscle weakness after exercise
Muscle stiffness
Muscle aches
Muscle cramps
Muscle contractions
Muscle spasms
Muscle tenderness
Pins and needles sensation
Eyelid myotonia

Digestion
Upset stomach
Loss of appetite
Vomiting
Constipation
Diarrhea
Bloating of the stomach
Full feeling in the stomach
Paralytic ileus

Heart
Anxiousness
Irregular and rapid heartbeat
Angina
Prominent U waves
Inverted or flattened T waves
ST depression
Elongated PR interval

Kidneys
Severe thirst
Increased urination
Difficulty breathing
Too slow or shallow breathing
Lack of oxygen in the blood
Sweating
Increased blood pressure
Metabolic acidosis

Liver
Irritability
Depression
Decrease in concentration
Lack of clear thinking
Confusion
Slurring of speech
Seizures

Paralysis
Episodic muscle weakness
Episodic partial paralysis
Episodic total paralysis
Episodic flaccid paralysis

Laboratory blood changes
Increased number of neutrophils in blood,
Increased number of white blood cells in the blood,
Reduced number of eosinophils in blood,
Increased number of lymphocytes in blood,
Low blood sodium,
Low blood potassium
Elevated Serum CPK (creatine)

Laboratory urine changes
Excess protein in urine
Excess sugar in the urine
Excessive acetone in urine
Presence of renal casts in urine

The Personal Periodic Paralysis Journal

Symptoms Of HyperPP, NormoPP, PMC And ATS (Typically)

(Circle or check those that apply)

Muscles
Fatigue
Weakness
Pins and needles
Tingling or numbness in the extremities
Muscle contraction
Muscle rigidity
Muscle cramps
Muscles stiffness
Muscle twitching
Muscle cramping
Reduced reflexes
Muscle contraction involving tongue
Tightness in legs
Strange feeling in legs

Digestion
Discomfort
Nausea
Vomiting
Stomach cramps
Diarrhea

Heart
Palpitations
Chest pain
Irregular heartbeat
Slow heartbeat
Weak pulse
Absent pulse
Heart stoppage
Small P waves
Tall T waves
QRS abnormality
P wave abnormality
Long QT
Fast heartbeat

Kidneys
Breathing problems
Wheezing
Shortness of breath
Fast breathing
Feeling hot
Low blood pressure

Liver
Irritability
Sleepiness
Confusion
Seizures
Loss of consciousness

Paralysis
Episodic muscle weakness
Episodic partial paralysis
Episodic total paralysis

Laboratory blood changes
Elevated blood potassium
Serum sodium level elevated
Elevated Serum CPK (creatine)

Laboratory urine changes
Elevated urine pH level

The Periodic Paralysis Guide And Workbook

Personal Medical History

(Circle or check those that apply)

NEUROLOGICAL
Fainting spells
Seizures
Amnesia
Dizziness
Headaches
Paralysis
Vertigo
Fatigue
Muscle weakness
Nervousness
Loss of strength
Falling
TIA
Stroke
Loss of consciousness
Numbness
Pins and needles
Neuropathy
Headaches
Migraines
Loss of feeling/sensation

RESPIRATORY
Shallow breathing
Hyperventilation
Irregular breathing
Cough
Sputum
Shortness of breath
Asthma
Low oxygen
Difficulty breathing
Weak breathing muscles

CARDIOVASCULAR
Chest pain
High blood pressure
Low blood pressure
Heart murmur
Irregular heartbeat
Heart attack
Stroke
Blood clot in lung
Ankle swelling
Bradycardia
Tachycardia
Heart monitor
Pacemaker
Defibrillator
Wheezing
Palpitations
Long QT

GASTROINTESTINAL
Nausea
Vomiting
Change in bowel habits
Distention
Tarry stools
Bloody stools
Diarrhea
Heartburn
GERD
Diverticulitis
Abdominal pain
Constipation
IBS

MUSCULOSKELETAL
Back pain
Neck pain
Leg pain
Arm pain
Fractures
Joint pain
Joint swelling
Stiffness
Stress fractures
Scoliosis
Kyphosis
Osteoporosis
Osteopenia
Degenerative disk disease
Osteoarthritis
Rheumatoid arthritis

EARS, EYES, NOSE & THROAT
Nose bleeds
Sinus drainage
Sore throat
Difficulty swallowing
Choking
Hearing loss
Vision loss

Cataracts
Macular degeneration
Glasses
Blurred vision
Double vision
Loss of vision
Dizziness
Ringing in ears
Ear infections

PROSTHESIS
(Do you have any of the following?)
Removable bridge
Artificial eye
Hearing aid
Pacemaker
Artificial limbs
Brace
Internal metal clips
Where? _____

URINARY SYSTEM
Frequency in urination
Burning on urination
Bloody urine.
Unable to control bladder

KIDNEY/RENAL
Kidney infections
Kidney stones
Renal Failure

GLANDS, HORMONES & SUGAR CONTROL
Diabetes
Insulin?
Hypoglycemia
Thyroid deficiency
Thyroid excess
Cold
Hot
Fatigue
Overweight
Underweight

METABOLIC/ELECTROLYTES
Hyperkalemia
Hypokalemia
Metabolic acidosis
Lactic acidosis
Sepsis
Magnesium hi/low
Chloride hi/low
Sodium hi/low

BLOOD & LYMPH NODES
Anemia
Swollen glands
Clotting issues
Bruise easy
Excessive bleeding

VASCULAR
Edema/water retention
Arteriosclerosis
Vein Distension
Blood clots

SKIN
Thin
Itchy
Rash
Loose/Stretchy
Tight
Dry
Oily

GENERAL
Sleeping problems
Fever
Weight gain
Weight loss

MENTAL/EMOTIONAL
Depression
Anxiety
Bi-polar
ADD
ADHD
Learning disability
PTSD
Behavior disorder
Autism

INFECTIOUS PROBLEMS
Frequent infections
Type? _____

REPRODUCTIVE
PMS
Endometriosis
Heavy flow
Cramps
Fibroid tumors
Hysterectomy
Prostrate problems

DENTAL/MOUTH
Dentures
Sores
Periodontal disease
TMJ
TMD
TMD
Dry mouth
Teeth missing at birth
Small mandible

ALLERGIES
Hives
Foods
Asthma
Insect bites
Medications
Hay fever
Animal
Latex
Rashes

Use the space below to list any information that may need an explanation.

_____
_____
_____
_____
_____
_____
_____
_____
_____
_____

Have you been diagnosed with allergies, autoimmune and/or inflammatory diseases?

ALLERGIES, AUTOIMMUNE & INFLAMMATORY DISEASES
(All Autoimmune)

AUTOIMMUNE DISEASES
Addison's disease
Alopecia areata
Ankylosing spondylitis
Autoimmune angioedema
Autoimmune aplastic anemia
Autoimmune dysautonomia
Autoimmune hepatitis
Autoimmune hyperlipidemia
Autoimmune immunodeficiency
Autoimmune inner ear disease
Autoimmune myocarditis
Autoimmune oophoritis
Autoimmune pancreatitis
Autoimmune retinopathy
Autoimmune thrombocytopenic purpura
Autoimmune thyroid disease
Autoimmune urticaria
Axonal & neuronal neuropathies
Behcet's disease
Cardiomyopathy
Celiac disease
Chronic fatigue syndrome
Chronic inflammatory demyelinating Polyneuropathy
Chronic recurrent multifocal ostomyelitis
Crohn's disease
Congenital heart block
CREST disease
Demyelinating neuropathies
Dermatomyositis
Discoid lupus
Dressler's syndrome
Endometriosis
Fibromyalgia
Glomerulonephritis
Goodpasture's syndrome
Graves' disease
Guillain-Barre syndrome
Hashimoto's encephalitis

Hashimoto's thyroiditis
Hemolytic anemia
Immunoregulatory lipoproteins
Inclusion body myositis
Interstitial cystitis
Juvenile arthritis
Juvenile diabetes (Type 1 diabetes)
Juvenile myositis
Kawasaki syndrome
Lambert-Eaton syndrome
Lichen planus
Lichen sclerosus
Lupus
Lyme disease, chronic
Meniere's disease
Mixed connective tissue disease
Multiple sclerosis
Myasthenia gravis
Myositis
Narcolepsy
Neutropenia
Optic neuritis
Peripheral neuropathy
Pernicious anemia
Polymyalgia rheumatica
Polymyositis
Progesterone dermatitis
Primary biliary cirrhosis
Psoriasis
Psoriatic arthritis
Idiopathic pulmonary fibrosis
Raynauds phenomenon
Reactive Arthritis
Reflex sympathetic dystrophy
Reiter's syndrome
Relapsing polychondritis
Restless legs syndrome
Rheumatic fever
Rheumatoid arthritis
Sarcoidosis
Scleroderma
Sjogren's syndrome
Stiff person syndrome
Subacute bacterial endocarditis
Type I diabetes
Ulcerative colitis
Undifferentiated connective tissue dis.
Vasculitis

INFLAMMATORY DISEASES
ALS
Addison's disease
Aging (senescence)
Allergies and sensitivities
Anemia
Ankylosing spondylitis
Anorexia and bulimia
Anxiety
Asthma
Autism spectrum disorder
Baldness (alopecia)
Bipolar Disorder (manic-depression)
Cancer
Cardiovascular diseases
Cat scratch fever
Celiac disease
Chronic Lyme disease
Chronic fatigue syndrome
Co-infections
Cognitive dysfunction (brain fog)
Depression
Diabetes, Type II
Epilepsy (seizures)
Eye diseases
Fibromyalgia
Graves' disease
Hashimoto's disease
Headaches and migraines
Hypercalcemia
Hypertension (high blood pressure)
Inflammatory bowel disease (Crohn's disease and ulcerative colitis)
Irritable bowel
Kidney disease
Kidney stones
Learning disabilities (ADHD, ADD, dyslexia)
Mental and neurological conditions
Multiple chemical sensitivity
Multiple sclerosis
Obesity
Obsessive-compulsive disorder
Osteoarthritis
Osteoporosis and osteopenia
Parkinson's disease
Periodontal disease and gingivitis
Peripheral neuropathy
Pernicious anemia
Psoriasis
Raynaud's syndrome
Reiter's syndrome
Restless leg syndrome
Rheumatoid arthritis
Sarcoidosis
Schizophrenia
Scleroderma
Secondary hyperparathyroidism
Systemic lupus erythematosus
Cystic fibrosis
Diabetes, Type I
HIV and AIDS
Rickets

Use the space below to list any other not listed.

_____
_____
_____
_____
_____
_____
_____
_____
_____
_____
_____
_____
_____
_____
_____
_____
_____
_____
_____
_____
_____
_____
_____
_____
_____
_____

The Personal Periodic Paralysis Journal

Have you been diagnosed with a Chromosome 17 condition?

CHROMOSOME 17 CONDITIONS (Some)
Alexander disease
Andersen-Tawil syndrome
Autoimmune Addison disease
Caffey disease
Canavan disease
Charcot-Marie-Tooth disease
Common variable immune deficiency
Congenital myasthenic syndrome
Cystinosis
Ehlers-Danlos syndrome
Familial atrial fibrillation
Fanconi anemia
Glycogen storage disease type I
Hereditary neuralgic amyotrophy
Hereditary neuropathy with liability to pressure palsies
Hyperkalemic periodic paralysis
Hypokalemic periodic paralysis
Job syndrome
Limb-girdle muscular dystrophy
Neuroblastoma
Neurofibromatosis type 1
Osteogenesis imperfecta
Paramyotonia congenita
Pompe disease
Potassium-aggravated myotonia
Progressive supranuclear palsy
Pseudohypoaldosteronism type 2
Psoriatic arthritis
Renal tubular dysgenesis
Short QT syndrome
Sjögren-Larsson syndrome
SOST-related sclerosing bone dysplasia
Spondylocostal dysostosis
Tarsal-carpal coalition syndrome
Usher syndrome

Use the space below to list any other not listed.

_____
_____
_____
_____

CHARACTERISTICS OF ATS
Widely spaced eyes
Short stature
Scoliosis
Kyphosis
Webbed toes or fingers (partial or total between second and third toes)
Unusual short fingers
Long crooked fingers
Low set ears
Broad forehead
Small jaw
Protruding jaw
Receding jaw
Broad nasal root
Ventricular arrhythmia
Abnormal heart rhythm
Long QT interval heart beat
Irregular heartbeat
Discomfort
Fainting caused by irregular heartbeat
Dental abnormalities
Born with missing teeth
Late or non-loss of baby teeth
Low-set ears
Widely spaced eyes
Narrow set eyes
Abnormal curving of fingers (little fingers curve inward)
Abnormal curving of toes
Clubbed thumbs
Short opening for the eyes (between the eyelids)
Abnormal smallness of the head
Slowed degree of maturation of bones
Looseness of the muscles and soft tissue (surrounding a joint)
Small cheekbones
An abnormally low position (drooping) of the upper eyelid
Cleft palate
High arched palate
Mild learning difficulties
Distinct neuro-cognitive phenotype
Deficits in executive function
Deficits in abstract reasoning

Have you been diagnosed with a mitochondrial disease and/or do you have mitochondrial dysfunction?

MITOCHONDRIAL DISEASES
Alzheimer's Disease
Parkinson's' Disease
Ataxia, myoclonus and deafness
chronic intestinal pseudo obstruction with myopathy and ophthalmoplegia
Chronic Progressive External ophthalmoplegia
Cyclic Vomiting Syndrome
Maternally inherited deafness or Aminoglycoside-induced deafness
Dementia and chorea
Diabetes mellitus and deafness
Exercise intolerance
Epilepsy, strokes, optic atrophy and cognitive decline
Familial bilateral striatal necrosis
Fatal Infantile cardiomyopathy plus, a MELAS-associated cardiomyopathy
Gastrointestinal reflux
Kearns Sayre Syndrome
Leber's Hereditary Optic Neuropathy and Dystonia
Leber Hereditary Optic Neuropathy
Lethal Infantile Mitochondrial Myopathy
Myopathy and Diabetes Mellitus
Mitochondrial Encephalomyopathy, Lactic acidosis and stroke-like episodes
Myoclonic epilepsy and psychomotor regression
Myoclonic epilepsy and ragged red muscle fibers
Maternally inherited diabetes and deafness
Maternally Inherited hypertrophic cardiomyopathy
Maternally inherited cardiomyopathy
Maternally Inherited Leigh Syndrome
Mitochondrial encephalocardiomyopathy
Mitochondrial encephalomyopathy
Mitochondrial myopathy
Maternal myopathy and cardiomyopathy
Multisystem Mitochondrial Disorder (myopathy, encephalopathy, blindness, hearing loss, peripheral neuropathy)
Neurogenic muscle weakness, Ataxia, and Retinitis Pigmentosa; alternate phenotype at this locus is reported as Leigh Disease
Non-Insulin Dependent Diabetes Mellitus
Progressive Encephalopathy
Progressive Myoclonus Epilepsy
Rett Syndrome
Sudden Infant Death Syndrome
Sensorineural hearing loss

MITOCHONDRIAL DYSFUNCTION
Cancers (some)
Exercise intolerance
Strokes
Seizures
Gastrointestinal problems (reflux, vomiting, constipation, diarrhea)
Swallowing difficulties
Failure to thrive
Blindness
Deafness
Heart and kidney problems
Muscle failure
Heat/cold intolerance
Diabetes
Lactic acidosis
Immune system problems
Liver disease

Use the space below to list any other not listed.
_____
_____
_____
_____
_____

Tests Related To Periodic Paralysis

Test	Date	Results
Genetic DNA		
Whole Genome		
Muscle Biopsy		
CMAP		
Sleep Study		
Muscle Strength		
Oximeter/Oxygen		
Heart Stress		
Holter Monitor		
Holter Monitor		
Holter Monitor		
EKG/ECG		
EKG/ECG		
EKG/ECG		
EMG		
EMG		
EMG		
Nerve Conduction		
Nerve Conduction		
Nerve Conduction		
A1c Blood Sugar		
A1c Blood Sugar		
A1c Blood Sugar		
Creatinine		
Creatinine		
D-dimmer		
Potassium		
Potassium		
Potassium		

Tests Ruling Everything Else Out

Test	Date	Results
Chromosomal		
Metabolic		
MRI Spine		
MRI Brain		
Cat Scan		
Spinal Tap		
Upper GI		
Colonoscopy		
X-rays		
X-rays		
X-rays		
Blood Gases		
Allergies		
Arthritis		
Endocrine		
Bone Scan		
Hearing		
Vision		
Kidney		
Iron/Anemia		
Lungs		
Respiratory		
Ear, Nose, Throat		
ADD/ADHD		
Learning Disorder		
Cholesterol		
Neurological Exam		

The Personal Periodic Paralysis Journal

Triggers Chart
(Circle those that apply)

HYPOPP TRIGGERS
Large carbohydrate meal
Drinking alcohol
Ingesting too much salt
Stress (good or bad)
Excitement
Fear
Vigorous exercise
Resting after exercise
Cold
Epinephrine/adrenaline
Cold
Anesthesia

HYPERPP TRIGGERS
Large carbohydrate meal
Exercise
Cold
Ingesting too much potassium
Stress (good or bad)
Rest after exercise
Fatigue
Fasting
Cigarette smoke

PMC TRIGGERS
Exercise
Exertion
Repetitious movement
Cold
Sleeping in

GENERAL PP TRIGGERS
Diet:
Simple carbohydrates:
Sugar
White flour
Other
Complex carbohydrates:
Some grains
Wheat
Rye
Oats
Other

Meat:
Mostly red meats

Salt
Caffeine
MSG
Alcohol
Large meals
Gluten

Sleep:
All aspects of sleep:
Falling asleep
During sleep
Waking up

Other:
Dehydration
Fasting
Sitting too long
Changes in the weather
Fatigue
Heat
Cold
Electromagnetic Force (EMF's)
Menstrual cycle

Exercise

Rest after exercise

Unknown:

Over-the-counter medications
Cough syrups
Eye drops
Glycerin enemas
NSAID's

Compounds or Chemicals
Sodium Hydroxide
Edetate Disodium
Stearic Acid

They may be in the following:
Lotions
Oils
Hair dyes or colors
Antiperspirants
Enemas
Suppositories
Soaps
Shampoos
Shaving creams
Foams
Toothpastes
Deodorants
Beauty products
Skincare products
Cosmetic products
Bath salts
Emollients
Ointments
Creams
Hair sprays
Perfumes
Colognes
Powders
Gels
Oils
Tonics
Mousse

Drugs:
Saline drips,
Glucose Infusion
Corticosteroids
Muscle relaxers
Beta blockers
Tranquilizers
Pain killers (analgesics)
Antihistamines
Puffers for asthma
Antibiotics
Cough syrups
Eye drops to dilate eyes
Contrast dye for MRI's
Lidocaine
Anesthetics
Epinepherine
Adrenaline

Use the space below to list any other triggers not listed.

Immunization and Vaccination Chart

Type Of Vaccination	Date	Results Or Side Effects

Potassium

Do you use potassium?
_____

If no, why not?
_____
_____
_____
_____
_____

If yes, what type or types?
_____
_____
_____
_____

If yes, how much?
_____
_____

If yes, how often?
_____
_____
_____

If yes, how does it help?
_____
_____
_____
_____
_____

If yes, do you have any side effects or problems with it? Describe below.
_____
_____
_____
_____
_____
_____

Off-Label Periodic Paralysis Medications Presently Taking

Medication	Reason	Amounts	How Often	Side Effects
Diamox				
Acetazolamide				
Dichlorphenamide				
Spironolactone				
Triamterene				
Mexiletine				

Other Medications Presently Taking

Medication	Reason	Amounts	How Often	Side Effects

Other Medications Presently Taking

Medication	Reason	Amounts	How Often	Side Effects

Medications Used In The Past

Medication	Reason	Side Effects

Medications Used In The Past

Medication	Reason	Side Effects

Surgeries

Type of Surgery	Date	Reason	Outcome and/or Complications

Have you had any problems with anesthesia?
_____
_____

High fever?
_____
_____

Trouble placing the breathing tube?
_____
_____

Paralysis?
_____
_____

Take too long to come out of it?
_____
_____

Drop in blood pressure?
_____
_____

Problems with IV?
_____
_____

Diagnosis of Malignant Hyperthermia?
_____
_____

Hospitalizations (not Surgical)

Hospitalization	Date	Reason	Outcome and/or Complications

Hospitalizations (not Surgical)

Hospitalization	Date	Reason	Outcome and/or Complications

Emergency Room Visits

ER Visits	Date	Reason	Outcome and/or Complications

Emergency Room Visits

ER Visits	Date	Reason	Outcome and/or Complications

Description Of Treatment Received In The Emergency Room

The Personal Periodic Paralysis Journal

Dental Procedures

Dental Procedure	Dentist	Date	Results or Side Effects

Family Medical History

Children and grandchildren who also have symptoms of PP or who are diagnosed with a form of PP and/or other medical issues					
Children	Age	M/F	Diag Y/N	Type of PP	Present Health

Siblings and their children who also have symptoms of PP or who are diagnosed with a form of PP and/or other medical issues					
Siblings	Age	M/F	Diag Y/N	Type of PP	Present Health

Mother

Mother's health

Age	Diag Y/N	Type of PP	Present Health & Other Diagnoses	Age at Death	Cause of Death

Mother's siblings and their children who also have symptoms of PP or who are diagnosed with a form of PP and/or other medical issues

Siblings	Age	M/F	Diag Y/N	Type of PP	Present Health

Mother's mother's health					
Age	Diag Y/N	Type of PP	Present Health & Other Diagnoses	Age at Death	Cause of Death

Mother's father's health					
Age	Diag Y/N	Type of PP	Present Health & Other Diagnoses	Age at Death	Cause of Death

Father

Father's health					
Age	Diag Y/N	Type of PP	Present Health & Other Diagnoses	Age at Death	Cause of Death

Father's siblings and their children who also have symptoms of PP or who are diagnosed with a form of PP and/or other medical issues					
Siblings	Age	M/F	Diag Y/N	Type of PP	Present Health

The Personal Periodic Paralysis Journal

Father's mother's health					
Age	Diag Y/N	Type of PP	Present Health & Other Diagnoses	Age at Death	Cause of Death

Father's father's health					
Age	Diag Y/N	Type of PP	Present Health & Other Diagnoses	Age at Death	Cause of Death

List any other family medical issues

Doctors Chart

Name & Dates	Type	Address	Phone	Results

Doctors Chart

Name & Dates	Type	Address	Phone	Results

The Personal Periodic Paralysis Journal

Andersen-Tawil Syndrome-Like Flow Chart Duggins-Critchfield & Alexander-Stevenson Family

*Italics = Family members who are symptomatic or have some characteristics.

	Alexander Duggins & *Martha Critchfield Died at 38 of blood clotting disorder		Sanderson Alexander & Harriet Stevenson		GGreat Grandfathers & GGreat Grandmothers
*William Periods of Paralysis. Died at 59 from Paralysis and heart & Wife #1 Carrie				*William Periods of Paralysis. Died at 59 from Paralysis and heart & Wife #2 Mary	Great Grandfather & Great Grandmother
*Gr-Uncle #1 (No children) Died sudden heart	*Gr-Uncle #3 (No children) Died sudden heart	*Grandfather L. Sudden death due to heart age 67 & *Wife #1 Grandmother	*Gr-Aunt #1 (No children) Periodic Paralysis symptoms	*Gr-Uncle #4 Died 41-heart stopped during paralysis periods of weakness and paralysis heart palpitations	Grandfather & Great Uncles Great Aunt & Grandmother
*Gr-Uncle #2 Died sudden heart		*Lahiee (mother) *Sister #1 (aunt)			Mother Aunt
		*Grandfather L. & Wife #2 *Sister #2 (aunt)			Grandfather & Second wife Aunt
		*Grandfather L. & *Wife #3			Grandfather & Third wife
		*Sister #3 (aunt) *Sister #4 (aunt) *Sister #5 (aunt)			Aunt Aunt Aunt

The Periodic Paralysis Guide And Workbook

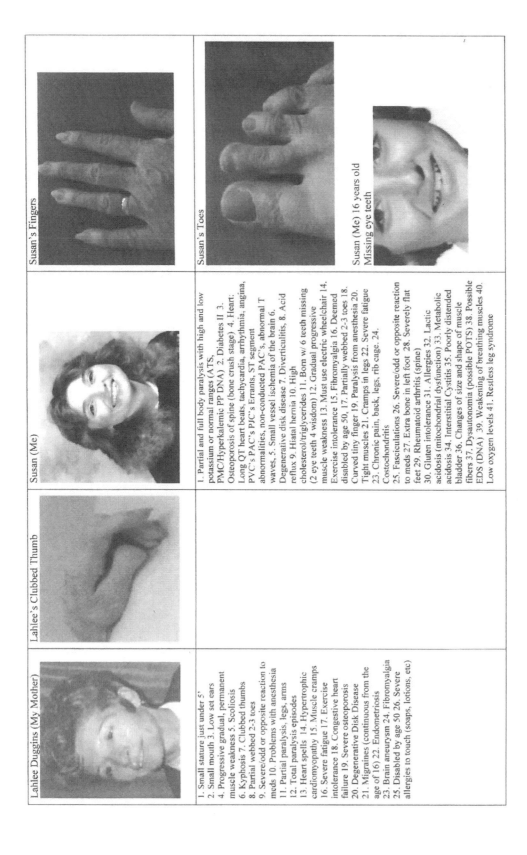

Lahlee Duggins (My Mother)	Lahlee's Clubbed Thumb	Susan (Me)	Susan's Fingers
			Susan's Toes
			Susan (Me) 16 years old Missing eye teeth
1. Small stature just under 5' 2. Small mouth 3. Low set ears 4. Progressive gradual, permanent muscle weakness 5. Scoliosis 6. Kyphosis 7. Clubbed thumbs 8. Partial webbed 2-3 toes 9. Severe/odd or opposite reaction to meds 10. Problems with anesthesia 11. Partial paralysis, legs, arms 12. Total paralysis episodes 13. Heart spells 14. Hypertrophic cardiomyopathy 15. Muscle cramps 16. Severe fatigue 17. Exercise intolerance 18. Congestive heart failure 19. Severe osteoporosis 20. Degenerative Disk Disease 21. Migraines (continuous from the age of 16) 22. Endometriosis 23. Brain aneurysm 24. Fibromyalgia 25. Disabled by age 50 26. Severe allergies to touch (soaps, lotions, etc)		1. Partial and full body paralysis with high and low potassium or normal ranges (ATS, PMC/Hyperkalemic PP DNA) 2. Diabetes II 3. Osteoporosis of spine (bone crush stage) 4. Heart: Long QT heart beats, tachycardia, arrhythmia, angina, PVC's PAC's PJC's Errants, ST segment abnormalities, non-conducted PAC's, abnormal T waves. 5. Small vessel ischemia of the brain 6. Degenerative disk disease 7. Diverticulitis, 8. Acid reflux 9. Hiatal hernia 10. High cholesterol/triglycerides 11. Born w/ 6 teeth missing (2 eye teeth 4 wisdom) 12. Gradual progressive muscle weakness 13. Must use electric wheelchair 14. Exercise intolerance 15. Fibromyalgia 16. Deemed disabled by age 50, 17. Partially webbed 2-3 toes 18. Curved tiny finger 19. Paralysis from anesthesia 20. Tight muscles 21. Cramps in legs 22. Severe fatigue 23. Chronic pain, back, legs, rib cage. 24. Costochondritis 25. Fasciculations 26. Severe/odd or opposite reaction to meds 27. Extra bone in left foot 28. Severely flat feet 29. Rheumatoid arthritis (spine) 30. Gluten intolerance 31. Allergies 32. Lactic acidosis (mitochondrial dysfunction) 33. Metabolic acidosis 34. Interstitial Cystitis 35. Poorly distended bladder 36. Changes of size and shape of muscle fibers 37. Dysautonomia (possible POTS) 38. Possible EDS (DNA) 39. Weakening of breathing muscles 40. Low oxygen levels 41. Restless leg syndrome	

Index

A
Abortive attacks: 7, 55
Acetazolamide: 25, 27, 31, 32, 89
Acidosis: , 9, 22, 24, 25, 26, 27, 28, 30, 31, 32, 35, 39, 61, 88, 93, 94, 105, 106, 124, 129, 134, 142, 152, 155, 160
    Lactic acidosis: 22, 25, 26, 27, 28, 35, 39, 129
    Metabolic acidosis: 9, 22, 24, 25, 26, 27, 28, 30, 31, 35, 61, 88, 93, 94, 105, 106, 129, 134, 142
Adrenaline (epinepherine): 10, 33, 59, 76, 85, 90, 104, 163
Alkaline (see pH levels): 26, 27, 93, 94, 95, 96, 98
Alkaline diet (pH balance diet): 93, 96, 98
Ambulance: 59, 60, 61, 62, 106, 123, 129, 131, 133, 134, 135, 136, 137, 138
Ambulance (when to call): 106, 131
Andersen-Tawil Syndrome: v, 6, 8, 12, 13, 15, 17, 23, 24, 28, 30, 33, 37, 39, 40, 45, 53, 54, 71, 103, 104, 107, 109, 111, 112, 115, 118, 120, 134, 135, 138
    Characteristics: 12, 13, 40
    Description: 6, 12
    Diagnosis: 12
    Prognosis: 12
    Symptoms: 12
    Treatment: 12
    Triggers: 12
Andersen-Tawil Syndrome-like: 40
Anesthesia: 13, 32, 33, 76, 163
Arrhythmia: 6, 12, 13, 22, 23, 25, 29, 32, 33, 36, 37, 38, 40, 43, 53, 54, 59, 61, 62, 106, 119, 123, 125, 128, 134, 137, 138, 159
    Long QT: 12, 13, 23, 25, 33, 36, 37, 39, 40, 54, 65, 71, 78, 88, 122, 129, 134, 136, 138, 139, 153, 154, 159
Palpatations: 174
    Torsades de pointes: 23, 33, 78
Attacks (see episodes): 1, 4, 5, 6, 7, 8, 9, 10, 11, 13, 14, 15, 20, 22, 23, 28, 29, 32, 33, 37, 38, 41, 42, 43, 45, 49, 53, 54, 55, 56, 57, 59, 65, 71, 77, 81, 84, 85, 87, 90, 93, 94, 95, 103, 106, 107, 108, 112, 116, 117, 118, 119, 123, 124, 128, 130, 134, 139, 141, 148, 160
Autoimmune diseases: 36

B
Balanced diet: 14, 46, 87, 93, 94, 95, 96, 141
Blood: ix, 5, 9, 10, 11, 17, 21, 22, 26, 27, 28, 30, 33, 34, 35, 37, 38, 40, 41, 43, 45, 53, 54, 55, 59, 60, 61, 62, 65, 74, 75, 88, 90, 104, 105, 106, 107, 117, 119, 123, 126, 128, 129, 131, 132, 134, 137, 138, 152, 153, 154, 158, 173
Blood draw (see tourniquet:) 117
Blood pressure: 9, 11, 21, 27, 30, 32, 37, 38, 41, 43, 45, 55, 59, 60, 62, 65, 74, 75, 88, 90, 104, 106, 107, 119, 123, 128, 134, 137, 152, 153, 154, 158, 173
Blood pressure cuff: 62, 65

Blood serum levels (see potassium levels): 2, 3, 5, 7, 8, 9, 10, 11, 12, 15, 22, 29, 32, 33, 34, 39, 40, 41, 53, 54, 59, 60, 65, 67, 104, 105, 106, 116, 117, 118, 132, 134
Blood sugar (see glucose)
Bradycardia (slow heartbeat) (see heart issues): 11, 22, 23
Breathing issues: 11, 24, 74, 75, 106, 121, 123, 154
    Carbon dioxide: 24, 26
Elephant on chest: 106
Hyperventilation (see fast breathing): 27, 75
Hypoventilation (see slow breathing): 24, 27, 118
Weak breathing muscles: 24, 28
Oxygen: 9, 21, 24, 25, 27, 28, 35, 46, 59, 60, 61, 85, 87, 93, 103, 104, 106, 107, 109, 112, 116, 117, 119, 124, 128, 129, 130, 134, 141, 152, 154
Oxygen levels: 24, 25, 27, 28, 60, 61, 106, 107, 120
Respiratory arrest/failure: 24, 59, 71, 106
Breathing muscles: 14, 24, 25, 27, 28, 71, 124, 154
Breathing stops: 106

C
CACNA1C: 6
CACNA1S: 6, 29
Cardiac arrest: 22, 23, 25, 53, 59, 71, 139
Cardy meter (see tools): 10, 11, 53, 60, 61, 105, 129
Channelopathy (see ion channelopathy)
Characteristics (see Andersen-Tawil Syndrome): 3, 6, 7, 12, 13, 30, 37, 38, 40, 43, 115, 118, 119, 125, 126, 130, 145
    Andersen-Tawil Syndrome-like characterisitcs: 107
Chest pain (see heart issues/angina)
Choking: 7, 32, 37, 38, 43, 53, 56, 59, 106, 107, 134, 137
Cold: 7, 10, 11, 14, 27, 35, 46, 59, 75, 83, 87, 90, 105, 160
Complications: 19, 20, 22, 23, 27, 33, 34, 35, 36, 38, 39, 40, 42, 43, 59, 71, 88, 93, 108, 119, 129, 139
    Co-existing Complications: 35, 36, 37, 38, 111, 147
Conversion disorder: 18, 30, 41, 42, 43, 109, 112, 115, 124, 127, 129, 132
Criteria for making genetic diagnosis: 6

D
Death: 17, 23, 26, 27, 30, 31, 32, 33, 41, 42, 43, 71, 88, 89, 95, 106, 118, 124, 125, 130, 138, 140, 142
Dehydration: 94, 103
Depression: 9, 21, 22, 35, 104, 124, 128, 152, 158
Diabetes: 35, 39, 61, 109, 112, 130, 136, 157, 160
Diagnosis: ix, x, 1, 2, 3, 4, 7, 17, 18, 20, 22, 23, 25, 28, 30, 31, 35, 36, 37, 38, 39, 41, 42, 43, 45, 49, 50, 63, 65, 85, 88, 109, 111, 112, 115, 116, 118, 119, 120, 123, 124, 125, 126, 127, 128, 129, 130, 131, 132, 134, 135, 136, 137, 141, 142, 143, 145, 146, 147
Clinical: 2, 3, 38, 115, 116, 119, 130, 147
Genetic: 3, 31, 38

Index

How to get: 115
New form/chart (Periodic Paralysis Plus 10 Syndrome (PP+10S): 39, 121, 122
Diamox (see acetazolamide): 25, 27, 31, 32, 89
Diet (see Alkaline diet)
Digestion: 9, 11, 17, 20
Discussion/support groups: 19, 21, 49, 51, 90, 92, 103, 104, 136, 137
Distilled water: 46, 87
DNA (see genetic mutations)
Doctors: ix, x, 1, 3, 18, 28, 30, 32, 42, 43, 45, 46, 47, 49, 60, 84, 85, 94, 106, 109, 110, 111, 112, 115, 116, 117, 118, 119, 120, 123, 126, 127, 128, 129, 130, 134, 135, 136, 138, 141, 142
    How to find: 109
    How to direct: 127, 135
    MDA: 111
    Primary Care (PCP): iii, 25, 47, 110, 111, 112, 116 127, 157,
Drugs (medications/pharmaceuticals): x, 4, 7, 9, 10, 11, 13, 14, 22, 24, 25, 26, 27, 28, 29, 30, 31, 32, 33, 35 36, 38, 39,41, 42, 43, 59, 61, 71, 76, 77, 78, 81, 83, 88, 89, 93, 94, 95, 105, 106, 109, 111, 112, 116, 118, 119, 123, 124, 125, 128, 129, 130, 131 134, 136, 137, 138, 139, 141, 142, 143, 148, 163

E
Educate Yourself: 49
Effective Functioning Disorder: 13
EMF: 77, 105, 163
Emergency chart: 131, 132, 133, 134, 135, 138
Emergency Room (see ER): viii, xii, 1, 32, 41, 43, 118, 119, 123, 129, 134, 135, 136, 139, 176, 177, 178
EKG: 22, 23, 26, 117, 119, 162
Endocrinologist: 18, 128
Epinepherine (see adrenaline): 10, 33, 59, 76, 85, 90, 104, 163
Episodes (attacks): 1, 4, 5, 6, 7, 8, 9, 10, 11, 13, 14, 15, 20, 22, 23, 28, 29, 32, 33, 37, 38, 41, 42, 43, 45, 49, 53, 54, 55, 56, 57, 59, 65, 71, 77, 81, 84, 85, 87, 90, 93, 94, 95, 103, 106, 107, 108, 112, 116, 117, 118, 119, 123, 124, 128, 130, 134, 139, 141, 148, 160
Episodes (types):
    Abortive: 7, 55
    Andersen-Tawil Syndrome: 7, 12, 13, 54, 55
    Description of: 53
    Falling (dropping): 2, 33, 45, 61, 75, 85, 100, 104, 106, 124
    Full-body (total): 39, 55, 120, 122, 137
    Hyperkalemic Periodic Paralysis: 5, 10, 54
    Hypokalemic Periodic Paralysis: 5, 9, 53
    Normokalemic Periodic Paralysis: 6, 13, 54
Paramyotonia Congenita: 6, 14, 54
Partial: 10, 11, 12, 24, 28, 37, 38, 39, 43, 53, 59, 71, 74, 75, 81, 87, 103, 117, 120, 122, 152, 153, 159

Throtoxic Periodic Paralysis: 6, 15, 55
Total (see full-body)
ER (Emergency Room): viii, xii, 1, 32, 41, 43, 118, 119, 123, 129, 134, 135, 136, 139, 176, 177, 178
Executive Function Disorder (AFD): 13
Exercise intolerance: 20, 21, 22, 25, 35, 38, 39, 77, 81, 93, 103, 104, 124, 126

F
Fainting (passing out/syncope): 23, 35, 53, 54
Falling: 65, 112
Fast heart rate (tachycardia): 7, 21, 22, 23, 24, 25, 26, 29, 37, 38, 54, 61, 71, 104, 128
Family: ix, 1, 2, 3, 4, 12, 14, 32, 43, 47, 49, 50, 59, 109, 110, 115, 118, 119, 124, 125, 130, 132, 135, 136, 143, 145, 186
Fibromyalgia: 28, 35, 36, 39
Friends: 49, 92, 109, 112, 124

G
G72.3: 131
Gamstorp Disease (see Hyperkalemic Periodic Paralysis): 10
Genetic mutations/codes (DNA):
    CACNA1C: 6
    CACNA1S: 6, 29
    KCNE3: 6
    KCNJ2: 6
    KCNJ5: 6
    KCNJ18: 6
    SCN4A: 6, 31, 36
Genetic diagnosis: 3, 31, 38
Genetic testing: x, 3, 111, 115, 116, 124, 125, 126, 142
Glucose (blood sugar): 32, 33, 41, 46, 87, 105, 119, 124, 133, 139

H
Heart arrhythmia (see arrhythmia/heart issues)
Heart issues (see arrhythmia)
    Angina (chest pain): 9, 11, 26, 28, 107
    Arrhythmia (irregular heartbeat): 6, 12, 13, 22, 23, 25, 29, 32, 33, 36, 37, 38, 40, 43, 53, 54, 59, 61, 62, 106, 119, 123, 125, 128, 134, 137, 138, 159
    Bradycardia (slow heartbeat): 11, 22, 23
    Long QT: 12, 13, 23, 25, 33, 36, 37, 39, 40, 54, 65, 71, 78, 88, 122, 129, 134, 136, 138, 139, 153, 154, 159
    Palpitations (see arrhythmia): 74
    Tachycardia (fast heartbeat): 7, 22, 23, 24, 25, 26, 29, 37, 38, 54, 61, 71, 128, 138
    Ventricular arrhythmia: 12, 40, 134
Heat: 7, 46, 56, 59, 87, 90, 105
High potassium (see hyperkalemia) (see potassium levels): 6, 8, 10, 11, 14, 22, 26, 41, 54, 96, 105, 106, 115, 116, 134

Index

Hospital: 1, 43, 59, 110, 123, 128, 129, 131, 134, 135, 136, 137, 138, 142
Hospital Staff: 135
    How to direct: 135
Hydration: 29
Hyperactivity: 13
Hyperkalemia (high potassium): 5, 8, 10, 23, 24, 26, 54, 105, 135
Hyperkalemic Periodic Paralysis (Gamstorp Disease): v, 6, 7, 8, 10, 11, 13, 14, 15, 22, 23, 28, 32, 33, 41, 54, 55, 71, 76, 78, 96, 103, 104, 105, 135
    Description: 5, 10
    Diagnosis: 11
    Prognosis: 11
    Symptoms: 11
    Treatment: 11
    Triggers: 11
Hyperventilation (see breathing issues): 27, 75
Hypochondriac (see psychiatric disorders): 13
Hypokalemia (low potassium): 5, 9, 22, 33, 53, 54, 134
Hypokalemic Periodic Paralysis (Westphall Disease): v, 6, 7, 9, 10, 13, 15, 22, 23, 28, 29, 31, 33, 36, 41, 49, 53, 54, 55, 71, 76, 96, 103, 104, 105, 135
    Description: 5, 9
    Diagnosis: 9
    Prognosis: 9
    Symptoms: 9
    Treatment: 9
    Triggers: 9
Hypoventilation: 24, 27, 118

I
Iatrogenic: 43, 123, 129, 130
Imagery (meditation): 87, 92, 107
Incurable (see prognosis): 20, 93
Individualization: 4
Internet: 135
Ion channelopathies: 4, 5, 17, 18, 32, 36, 38 117, 119
Irregular heartbeat (see arrhythmia)
IV's: viii, 32, 41, 43, 78, 88, 123
    Glucose (dextrose, sugar): 32, 78
        Hartmann's IV Solution: 32, 78
        Mannitol: 32, 78
        Saline (sodium, salt): 32, 78

J
Journal (Personal Periodic Paralysis Journal): vii, 92, 101, 128, 145, 147

K
KCNE3: 6
KCNJ2: 6
KCNJ5: 6
KCNJ18: 6
Kidney: 9, 11, 25, 26, 29, 31, 35, 124, 128, 129, 139, 142, 160
Kidney (hyperkalemia): 11
Kidney (hypokalemia): 9
Kidney stones: 25, 26, 31, 35, 124, 129, 142

L
Laboratory changes: 10, 11
Laboratory changes (hyperkalemia): 11
Laboratory changes (hypokalemia): 10
Lactic acidosis (see acidosis): 22, 25, 26, 27, 28, 35, 39, 129
Learning disabilities: 13
Lidocaine (see anesthesia): 20, 33
Lifestyle changes: 143
Liver: 10, 11
Liver (hyperkalemia): 11
Liver (hypokalemia): 10
Long QT heartbeat (see arrhythmia): 12, 13, 23, 25, 33, 36, 37, 39, 40, 54, 65, 71, 78, 88, 122, 129, 134, 136, 138, 139, 153, 154, 159
Low potassium (see hypokalemia) (see potassium levels): 5, 9, 22, 33, 53, 54, 134

M
Malingerer: (see psychiatric disorders)
Malignant Hyperthermia: 32, 33, 36, 123
Management of Periodic Paralysis (see treatment)
MDA (Muscular Dystrophy Association): 18, 46, 47, 109, 111, 112, 127, 147
MDA doctors: 111
Medications (drugs): x, 4, 7, 9, 10, 11, 13, 14, 22, 24, 25, 26, 27, 28, 29, 30, 31, 32, 33, 35 36, 38, 39, 41, 42, 43, 59, 61, 71, 76, 77, 78, 81, 83, 88, 89, 93, 94, 95, 105, 106, 109, 111, 112, 116, 118, 119, 123, 124, 125, 128, 129, 130, 131 134, 136, 137, 138, 139, 141, 142, 143, 148, 163
    Adverse effects: 29, 129
    Cause of Long QT: 78
    Cause of Torsades de pointes: 78
    Idiosyncratic effect: 29, 30, 31, 88, 89, 123
    Over-the-counter: 77
    Paradoxical effect: 29, 35
    Side effects: (see adverse effects)
Meditation: 46, 87
Mentally ill (see psychiatric disorders):
Metabolic acidosis (see acidosis): 9, 22, 24, 25, 26, 27, 28, 29, 30, 31, 35, 61, 88, 89, 93, 94, 105, 106, 129, 134, 142

Index

Metabolic disorders: iii, x, xii, 1, 5, 17, 25, 30, 31, 32, 36, 59, 61, 88, 95, 96, 119, 130, 141

Mineral metabolic disorder: iii, x, xii, 1, 5, 17, 25, 30, 31, 32, 36, 59, 61, 88, 95, 96, 119, 130, 141

Mitochondrial disease: 20, 159

Monitor vitals: 59
    How to: 59
    When to: 59
    Why: 59
    Tools for (see tools):

MRI: 20, 78, 116, 119, 162, 164

Muscle biopsy: 20, 43, 119

Muscle myopathy: 19, 20, 21, 103, 160

Muscle symptoms:
    Hyperkalemia: 11
    Hypokalemia: 9

Muscle tightness: 14

Muscle twitching (fasciculations): 11, 75

Muscle wasting: 18, 19, 20, 22, 29, 71

Muscle weakness: 7, 9, 10, 11, 14, 17, 19, 20, 26, 31, 32, 36, 39, 42, 43, 55, 59, 71, 72, 74, 75, 77, 78, 81, 85, 87, 103, 115, 117, 120, 122, 124, 126, 128, 129, 136, 152, 153, 160

Muscle weakness (permanent): 14, 20, 31, 36, 42, 55, 103, 124, 126

Muscle weakness (progressive): 19, 20, 39

Muscular dystrophy: 18, 36, 111

Myopathy (see muscle myopathy)

N

Neurologist: ix, 18, 111, 116, 128, 147

Normal potassium level (see potassium levels): 12, 39, 40, 67

Normokalemia (normal potassium levels): 12, 39, 40, 67

Normokalemic dilemma: 40

Normokalemic Periodic Paralysis: 19
    Description: 19
    Diagnosis: 19
    Prognosis: 19
    Symptoms: 19
    Treatment: 19
    Triggers: 19

O

Obsessive-compulsive disorder: 13

Organic foods: 46, 87

Osteoporosis: 25, 26, 31, 35, 53, 71, 85, 124, 142

Over-the-counter medications (see medications)

Oximeter (see tools)

Oxygen (see breathing issues)

P

Pain: viii, 9, 11, 14, 21, 26, 27, 28, 29, 32, 42, 61, 75, 103, 104, 107, 109, 123, 137, 139, 153, 154

Paradoxical effect (see medications)

Paralysis:

Partial: 10, 11, 12, 24, 28, 37, 38, 39, 43, 53, 59, 71, 74, 75, 81, 87, 103, 117, 120, 122, 152, 153, 159

Total (whole-body): 39, 55, 120, 122, 137

Paralytic Attacks (see episodes):

Paramedics: 106, 129, 131, 132, 134, 135, 137, 138

Paramyotonia Congenita (Von Eulenberg's Disease): 20

Passing out (see fainting)

Periodic Paralysis: iii, iv, v, vi, vii, viii, ix, x, xi, xii, 1, 2, 3, 4, 5, 6, 7, 8, 9, 10, 11, 12, 13, 14, 15, 17, 18, 19, 20, 21, 22, 23, 24, 25, 26, 27, 28, 29, 30, 31, 32, 33, 34, 35, 36, 37, 38, 39, 40, 41, 42, 43, 45, 49, 50, 51, 53, 54, 55, 59, 60, 61, 62, 71, 72, 74, 76, 77, 78, 80, 82, 85, 87, 88, 89, 90, 93, 94, 95, 96, 98, 100, 103, 104, 105, 106, 108, 109, 110, 111, 112, 115, 117, 118, 119, 120, 122, 123, 124, 125, 126, 127, 128, 129, 130, 131, 132, 134, 135, 136, 137, 139, 140, 141, 142, 143, 145, 146, 147, 161, 167

    Description: 5

    Diagnosis: i, ix, x, 1, 2, 3, 4, 7, 17, 18, 20, 22, 23, 25, 28, 30, 31, 35, 36, 37, 38, 39, 41, 42, 43, 45, 49, 50, 63, 65, 85, 88, 109, 111, 112, 115, 116, 118, 119, 120, 123, 124, 125, 126, 127, 128, 129, 130, 131, 132, 134, 135, 136, 137, 141, 142, 143, 145, 146, 147

    Forms/types: 5, 9, 55

    Prognosis: 118

    Symptoms: i, x, xi, xii, 1, 2, 3, 4, 5, 6, 7, 8, 9, 10, 11, 13, 14, 15, 18, 19, 20, 21, 22, 23, 25, 26, 27, 29, 30, 31, 32, 33, 35, 36, 37, 38, 39, 40, 41, 43, 45, 46, 47, 49, 50, 53, 54, 55, 56, 57, 59, 60, 71, 72, 74, 78, 81, 83, 84, 85, 87, 88, 90, 92, 94, 95, 103, 104, 105, 107, 108, 109, 111, 112, 115, 116, 117, 118, 119, 120, 123, 124, 125, 126, 127, 128, 129, 130, 134, 136, 137, 139, 140, 141, 142, 143, 145, 147, 181, 182, 184

    Treatment: i, viii, 7, 20, 22, 27, 28, 29, 47, 127, 178

    Triggers: 1, 5, 7, 8, 10, 11, 13, 14, 23, 29, 30, 31, 33, 42, 45, 46, 47, 54, 63, 71, 72, 76, 83, 84, 85, 87, 88, 90, 93, 94, 115, 117, 118, 119, 123, 128, 141, 164

Periodic Paralysis Network: i, iii, iv, v, vi, ix, x, 2, 35, 42, 49, 50, 51, 6280, 82, 94, 100, 106, 122, 130, 142, 143

Periodic Paralysis Network, Inc: i, ii, iii, iv, v, viii, ix, 2, 36, 43, 50, 51, 53, 64, 82, 84, 96, 102, 108, 125, 132, 144, 145

Periodic Paralysis Plus 10 Syndrome: 3, 37, 122

Periodic Paralysis (types/forms):

    Andersen-Tawil Syndrome: v, 6, 8, 12, 13, 15, 17, 23, 24, 28, 30, 33, 37, 39, 40, 45, 53, 54, 71, 103, 104, 107, 109, 111, 112, 115, 118, 120, 134, 135, 138

    Hyperkalemic Periodic Paralysis: v, 6, 7, 8, 10, 11, 13, 14, 15, 22, 23, 28, 32, 33, 41, 54, 55, 71, 76, 78, 96, 103, 104, 105, 135

    Hypokalemic Periodic Paralysis: v, 6, 7, 9, 10, 13, 15, 22, 23, 28, 29, 31, 33, 36, 41, 49, 53, 54, 55, 71, 76, 96, 103, 104, 105, 135

Index

    Normokalemic Periodic Paralysis: 6, 7, 13, 15, 19, 28, 33, 41, 54, 103, 104, 105, 134

    Paramyotonia Congenita: v, 6, 8, 14, 15, 28, 36, 39, 45, 54, 76, 104

    Throtoxic Periodic Paralysis: 6, 7, 15, 55

Permanent Muscle weakness (see muscle weakness)

pH balance: 26, 93, 94, 95, 98

pH balance diet (alkaline diet): 27, 28, 96

pH levels: 11, 74, 153

    Acid: 24, 26, 27, 93, 96, 106

    Alkaline: 26, 27, 93, 94, 95, 96, 98

pH meter: 61

pH strips: 61

Pharmaceuticals (see drugs): x, 4, 7, 9, 10, 11, 13, 14, 22, 24, 25, 26, 27, 28, 29, 30, 31, 32, 33, 35 36, 38, 39,41, 42, 43, 59, 61, 71, 76, 77, 78, 81, 83, 88, 89, 93, 94, 95, 105, 106, 109, 111, 112, 116, 118, 119, 123, 124, 125, 128, 129, 130, 131 134, 136, 137, 138, 139, 141, 142, 143, 148, 163

Physical exercise: i, 21, 46, 87, 103

Physical exertion: 103

Physical therapy: i, 20, 41, 103

Potassium: i, 2, 3, 4, 5, 6, 7, 8, 9, 10, 11, 12, 13, 14, 15, 17, 22, 24, 25, 26, 27, 28, 29, 31, 32, 33, 34, 36, 37, 38, 39, 40, 41, 43, 47, 53, 54, 59, 60, 61, 65, 67, 71, 76, 87, 90, 93, 95, 96, 100, 104, 105, 106, 115, 116, 117, 118, 119, 123, 124, 128, 132, 134, 148, 152, 153, 163, 16

Potassium forms: 106

    Liquid: 106

    Powder: 106

    Salts: 106

    Tablets: 106

Potassium levels: 2, 3, 5, 7, 8, 9, 10, 11, 12, 15, 22, 29, 32, 33, 34, 39, 40, 41, 53, 54, 59, 60, 65, 67, 104, 105, 106, 116, 117, 118, 132, 134

    High: 6, 8, 10, 11, 14, 22, 26, 41, 54, 96, 105, 106, 115, 116, 134

    Low: 6, 15, 29, 32, 41, 53, 60, 96, 105, 116, 118

    Normal: 12, 39, 40, 67

    Speed of: 7, 53

Potassium reader: 10, 11, 53, 60, 61, 105, 129

Potassium shifting: 4, 6, 8, 13, 14, 24, 25, 26, 27, 28, 33, 36, 37, 38, 41, 42, 43, 71, 93, 104, 115, 116, 117, 118, 124

    Cause (see triggers)

    Results of (see episodes)

Potassium types (see potassium forms)

Prescriptions (see medications, drugs, pharmaceuticals)

Prognosis: viii, 118, 139

    Andersen-Tawil Syndrome: 12

    Death/deadly: 17, 20, 23, 26, 27, 30, 31, 32, 33, 41, 42, 43, 71, 88, 89, 95, 106, 118, 124, 125, 130, 138, 140, 142

    Hyperkalemic Periodic Paralysis: 11

    Hypokalemic Periodic: 9
    Incurable/no known cure: ix, x, 20, 142, 143
    Life-threatening: 7, 12, 22, 33, 40, 41, 42, 59, 71, 93, 123, 130, 134
    Normokalemic Periodic Paralysis: 19
    Paramyotonia Congenita: 20
    Periodic Paralysis: 139
    Sudden death: 23, 71
    Terminal: 20, 23
    Throtoxic Periodic Paralysis: 15
Progressive muscle weakness: 19, 20, 39
Psychiatric disorders (mentally ill): 132
    Conversion disorder: 18, 30, 41, 42, 43, 109, 112, 115, 124, 127, 129, 132
    Malingerer: 132
    Hypochondriac: 132
    Pseudo-seizures: 132

R
Respiratory arrest: (see breathing issues)
Rest: 10, 11, 21, 24, 29, 85, 103, 139
Restless leg syndrome: i, 35, 39, 53, 71
Rhabdomyolysis: 29

S
SCN4A: i, 6, 31, 36
Seizures: 10, 11, 35, 36, 41, 43, 134, 158
Seizure-like: 88
Slow heartbeat (see bradycardia): 11, 22, 23
Specialists: ix, xi 2, 4, 36, 109, 110, 111, 112, 124, 127, 128, 129, 130, 139, 141, 142, 144, 148
Speech (issue/difficulty): 10, 21, 55, 104, 152
Stress: 10, 11, 31, 35, 59, 71, 87, 90, 92, 94, 98, 100, 103, 119, 139, 143
    As triggers: 76
    Avoiding: 90
Sudden death (see prognosis): 23, 71
Supplements: 46, 87, 93, 100, 106, 142
Supplies (see tools)
Survey: 2, 3, 15, 35, 36, 37, 38, 40, 41
Swallowing: 20, 35, 71, 134, 154
Symptoms: x, xi, xii, 1, 2, 3, 4, 5, 6, 7, 8, 9, 10, 11, 13, 14, 15, 18, 19, 20, 21, 22, 23, 25, 26, 27, 29, 30, 31, 33, 35, 36, 37, 38, 39, 40, 41, 42, 43, 46, 47, 48, 50, 51, 55, 56, 57, 58, 59, 62, 63, 74, 75, 78, 82, 85, 87, 88, 89, 91, 92, 94, 96, 98, 99, 107, 108, 109, 111, 112, 113, 115, 116, 119, 120, 121, 122, 123, 124, 127, 128, 129, 130, 131, 132, 133, 134, 138, 140, 141, 143, 144, 145, 146, 147, 149, 151, 185, 186, 188
    Andersen-Tawil Syndrome: 12
    Hyperkalemic Periodic Paralysis: 11
    Hypokalemic Periodic Paralysis: 9

Index

Normokalemic Periodic Paralysis: 19
Paramyotonia Congenita: 20
Throtoxic Periodic Paralysis: 15
Syncope (see fainting): 23, 35, 54

T
Tachycardia (see heart issues): 7, 22, 23, 24, 25, 26, 29, 37, 38, 54, 61, 71, 128, 138
Team (medical): 47, 127, 131, 135
    Assemble and direct: 127
Terminal (see prognosis): 20, 23
Thyrotoxic Periodic Paralysis: 15
Tools: 59
    Blood pressure cuff: 62
    Blood glucose (sugar) meter: 61
    Cardy meter (see potassium reader): 10, 11, 53, 60, 61, 105, 129
    Oximeter: 61
    PH meter/strips: 61
Potassium reader: 10, 11, 53, 60, 61, 105, 129
Stethoscope: 62
Thermometer: 62
Torsades de pointes (see arrhythmia): 23, 33, 78
Tourniquet (blood draw): 28, 34, 131, 132, 135, 138
Treatment/management for: 2, 9, 11, 12, 15, 18, 19, 21, 34, 35, 36, 37, 39, 40, 43, 44, 46, 50, 51, 64, 86, 88, 110, 112, 113, 119, 120, 124, 125, 126, 129, 131, 132, 133, 135, 136, 137, 138, 140, 142, 146
    Andersen-Tawil Syndrome: 12
    Diet: 93, 96, 98
    Hyperkalemic Periodic Paralysis: 11
    Hypokalemic Periodic Paralysis: 9
    Lactic acidosis: 28
    Metabolic acidosis: 27
    Normokalemic Periodic Paralysis: 19
    Paramyotonia Congenita: 20
    Throtoxic Periodic Paralysis: 15
Triggers: i, 5, 7, 8, 10, 11, 13, 14, 23, 29, 30, 31, 33, 42, 45, 46, 47, 54, 63, 71, 72, 76, 83, 84, 85, 87, 88, 90, 93, 94, 115, 117, 118, 119, 123, 128, 141, 164
    Evaluate Data: 83
    How to find/discover: 71
    How to avoid: 88
    Hyperkalemic Periodic Paralysis: 11
    Hypokalemic Periodic Paralysis: 9
    Lists of: 76
    Trigger chart: 80
    Why to avoid: 71

U
Unprocessed foods: 46, 87, 94, 100

V
Ventricular arrhythmia (see arrhythmia)
Vitals:
    Monitoring vitals: 59
Von Eulenberg's Disease: (see Paramyotonia Congenita): 14

W
Westphall Disease (see Hypokalemic Periodic Paralysis): 9

Notes

Notes

Notes

Notes

Made in the USA
Columbia, SC
21 September 2018